what does it
feel like to
die?

what does it feel like to die?

Inspiring New Insights into the Experience of Dying

JENNIE DEAR

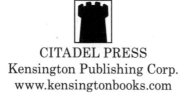

CITADEL PRESS
Kensington Publishing Corp.
www.kensingtonbooks.com

CITADEL PRESS BOOKS are published by

Kensington Publishing Corp.
119 West 40th Street
New York, NY 10018

Parts of "The Last Few Hours" and "Existential Slap" first appeared at TheAtlantic.com.

All Kensington titles, imprints, and distributed lines are available at special quantity discounts for bulk purchases for sales promotions, premiums, fund-raising, educational, or institutional use.

Special book excerpts or customized printings can also be created to fit specific needs. For details, write or phone the office of the Kensington sales manager: Kensington Publishing Corp., 119 West 40th Street, New York, NY 10018, attn: Sales Department; phone 1-800-221-2647.

CITADEL PRESS and the Citadel logo are Reg. U.S. Pat. & TM Off.

ISBN-13: 978-0-8065-3986-7
ISBN-10: 0-8065-3986-0

First Citadel trade paperback printing: July 2019

10 9 8 7 6 5 4 3 2 1

Printed in the United States of America

Library of Congress CIP data is available.

Electronic edition:

ISBN-13: 978-0-8065-3987-4 (e-book)
ISBN-10: 0-8065-3987-9 (e-book)

In memory of Martha Elizabeth Cannon Dear, who was not only intelligent, caring, and delightful, but also very private. I hope she would have forgiven me for writing so publicly about how she died.

In honor of the doctors, nurses, hospice workers and other medical professionals with whom I talked. Your interviews left me with a sense of wonder—at how much you give to your patients, and at your willingness to carve out time for me, for this book.

In honor of the hospice patients I've known, their patience or even their impatience; their love and sometimes their loneliness; their grief and even joy, as they encountered what we all will someday face.

author's note

Anyone who has been at the bedside of the dying has stories. Some are poignant, others are funny or angry or simply interesting; many are beautiful. A few of these appear in italicized sections interspersed through the book, in the words of the people who told them to me. Both in these sections and in the rest of the book, I've changed identifying details, substituted different names or used only initials to protect the privacy of patients and their family members.

contents

introduction

HERE'S WHAT I REMEMBER:

A hospice nurse sketching out logistics for my dying mother in terms both gentle and blunt. Then a pause, and the nurse asking, "Do you want to know what will happen as your body starts shutting down?"

She was offering to trace death's outlines on my mother's body, and to do that now, while my mother was mobile, coherent, and very much alive. There was a slight thrill of shock, of foreboding. But what my mother and I felt most strongly was relief, and something like fascination. We wanted to know.

Because, in the course of six and a half years of treatment, although my mother saw two general practitioners, six oncologists, a cardiologist, several radiation technicians, nurses at two chemotherapy facilities, and surgeons at three different clinics—not once, to my knowledge, had anyone talked to her about what would happen as she died.

This book originated in that moment with my mother and the hospice nurse, although it would be years before I left my job as an associate professor of English and journalism and started researching. In the meantime, I would become a hospice volunteer and I'd wonder about the patients I visited, too: What were they experiencing? When some patients' breaths began coming in strange noisy patterns in their last few hours, I wondered how much they were suffering, or whether it was possible they weren't suffering at all. I wondered why some people seemed in such deep denial about the fact that they were dying—as hospice patients, how could they not understand the implications? I was especially curious about where dying patients' minds were when they stopped responding to their families. I felt both concern and awe: Were they struggling deep inside with emotional or physical pain, or had they already embarked on an important spiritual journey?

As I began investigating, I was surprised to learn how much information there is about dying: research about pain and suffering, about how to cope with dying, about what the experience is like mentally and physically. Palliative care experts, hospice doctors, and nurses—anyone who spends time with dying people—have pondered many of the same questions I have. These people had the experience and expertise to study those questions in a scientific way, and they were producing academic papers, books, and articles about their work at an impressive rate. And most were willing to take time from hectic schedules to answer questions, in the hopes that more of that information might make its way to the general public.

Meanwhile, acquaintances or friends would ask what I was working on. When I replied that I was writing about dying, many would say some version of the following: "Oh, Americans do death so badly. We're a death-denying culture—nobody talks about death."

I didn't know quite how to take these comments, because it seems to me discussions about death are everywhere—think about how popular books like Atul Gawande's *Being Mortal* or Paul Kalanithi's *When Breath Becomes Air* have been, or the Pixar movie, *Coco,* or the hundreds of death cafés across the country created for the sole purpose of discussing death and dying.

Michelle Appenzeller, the clinical director at Hospice of Mercy in Durango, says the subject's current popularity sometimes strikes her as hilarious because it was such a taboo when she first began hospice work in 1986. "It's been so weird—funny, too," she says. "Death cafés, people wanting to talk about death—it's almost become cool and sexy." Still, my mother and I didn't know vital details until our conversation with the hospice nurse. Furthermore, all the discussion doesn't mean people are actually confronting their own deaths, says Appenzeller: "But still you can have a one-hundred-year-old, and you talk about hospice—and [the family is] shocked that their loved one's *dying.*"

The fact is, we talk about death and dying a lot in our culture, but that doesn't mean we face our own mortality, or that we talk enough about important aspects of dying, or that we have enough information about what dying is like. Most Americans don't have to deal with death directly as often or as soon in our lives as our ancestors did; and medical advances can feel so successful that we think they can fix anything. Many of us have lost touch with what dying is actually like. "Think about how people die on television or in the movies," says Marian Grant, a hospice and palliative care nurse practitioner and senior adviser to the Coalition to Transform Advanced Care. "They are awake to the end. They have meaningful conversations, and then their heads just turn to the side and . . . then they're dead."

But that image doesn't mirror reality. "That is not what any of this looks like," Grant says. "A hundred years ago, people died at home. People died in childbirth; children died. You would never have made it into adult life without having seen somebody you knew, a neighbor or someone in your community, actually die. Now, you could make it into your sixties or seventies and never have seen that. And what you see on television is this lovely romantic notion.

"But real life is *not* like that."

More than 90 percent of all Americans will almost certainly die as my mother did, living for weeks, months, or even years with the knowledge that they have a fatal disease. But most of us know little about what to expect during that time—despite the research from scholars on the experiences, symptoms, and emotional states of dying people, ranging from the "existential slap," the shattering realization after a fatal diagnosis that we really *are* mortal; to the amount of pain dying people endure; to the most successful methods in helping dying people cope. That knowledge still isn't widely available, despite a growing appetite for information about dying.

This book can't possibly treat all the information or all the facets of death and dying worth knowing about. My focus here is on what patients can expect to face in their final months. The book is based on research and interviews with doctors, nurses, psychologists, and other experts, and informed by my own deep sense of curiosity born from years of witnessing hospice patients' experiences. I've tried to be as honest as possible, even blunt sometimes, because that's what my mother and I craved when she was close to death. But I've also tried to convey some sense of the beauty and joy that often surround dying—the sense of meaning it can give to the dying person and people around her.

When one of my closest friends had septicemic plague, she said she wondered at one point whether she was dying (basically, she was, and she almost did, although she ultimately recovered). Then, she said, she realized she couldn't be—because she hadn't seen any Thestrals.

Thestrals, of course, are J.K. Rowling's imaginary creatures, skeletal horses with wings and dragon-like heads. It was only later, when my friend was better, that she realized her mistake: In Rowling's Harry Potter series, Thestrals are invisible to everyone except those who have witnessed someone else's death—they have nothing to do with your own death.

After my cousin died, his daughter told me she also came to appreciate the Thestrals. The fictional creatures were an apt metaphor for the way she now saw the world differently, and she suspected that Rowling must have experienced the death of someone close to her. As it turns out, Rowling had—her mother died at age forty-five when Rowling was just beginning to write her books.

It's telling that while the fictional characters who see Thestrals are saddened by their brush with death, their eyes have been opened.

chapter one

existential slap: a fatal diagnosis

The penalty we pay for believing that death comes only to other people is that it takes us by surprise.
—AVERY WEISMAN

I DON'T KNOW exactly when my mother, who eventually died of metastatic breast cancer, encountered her existential crisis. But I have a guess. My parents waited a day after her initial diagnosis before calling my brother, my sister, and me. They reached me first.

My father is not a terribly calm man, but he said, very calmly, something to this effect: "Your mother has been diagnosed with breast cancer."

There was a pause, and then a noise I can best describe as not quite a sob or a yell, but feral and animal-like. It was so uncharacteristic that I didn't know then, and I still don't know for certain, whether the sound came from my father or my mother.

I think that was the moment of her—and their—"existential slap," the instant when a person really comprehends, on a gut level, that death is close.

Palliative care pioneer Nessa Coyle coined the phrase to describe the experiences she witnessed in people with life-threatening illnesses. In her work as a nurse, Coyle noticed how tightly her patients clung to the belief that their diseases wouldn't kill them. She watched patients redefine what was most important in their lives, and what they hoped for as their health declined. Those changes in expectations were a process, something that happened over time. "But the actual realization that you're going to die, you're not going to beat this one—for many people, it seemed to me, came suddenly," she says. "Suddenly, they realized: *This is it.*"

Stephen was first diagnosed with prostate cancer in the early 1990s. The cancer was small and contained, so he decided against surgery or the relatively imprecise radiation treatments available at the time. Instead, he and his wife traveled to New York, San Diego, Los Angeles, and Scottsdale for a medley of treatments from leading prostate specialists and naturopaths. For years, the cancer remained stable, but it began to gradually spread and grow. Then, in 2013, Stephen's brother and son died within a week of each other, and his own health took a plunge. "I think that might have been the first glimpse of his own mortality, but I don't know that," says his wife, Jane. Stephen began seeking more aggressive treatments—radiation, an expensive medication prescribed by a doctor in California, a surgical procedure in Los Angeles. The disease continued to progress, and he continued to stave it off.

Then, in 2015, the couple made a memorable visit to the doctor's office: A gastroenterologist asked Stephen to lie down on the examination table. "He said, 'I think this is a tumor in your liver,'" Jane says. "And I remember the look on [Stephen]'s face. He was sitting there looking at me, and I was looking at him and he looked like a deer in the headlights. I'd never, ever seen that before . . . we just stared at each other. And I will always remember that."

While most people recognize on some level that death is inevitable, we don't really believe it, says Virginia Lee, a researcher and nurse who works with cancer patients: "At least in Western culture, we think we're going to live forever. We know on an intellectual level that we're not Superman, that we are not immortal. Kids learn that at an early stage, when pets die, or plants die, but that's at an intellectual level." Lee's patients often tell her they'd understood that death was real but thought of it as something that happened to other people—until they received their diagnosis. "The existential slap occurs when the reality and inevitability of one's own personal death sinks in," Coyle writes. "This awareness precipitates a crisis for most individuals."

Researchers have given the crisis other names: existential plight, or existential turning point. Crisis of knowledge of death. Ego chill. They say most patients with a terminal disease experience it, and it's not limited to one culture—people from different nations and different ethnicities have described it, although patients in places like the United States may be more susceptible simply because we have less exposure to death. The crisis can be terrifying and overwhelming. The moment of the existential slap usually happens, as it did for my mother, close to when doctors break the news.

"I've heard from cancer patients that your life changes instantly the moment the doctor or the oncologist says it's confirmed that it is cancer," Lee says. Doctors usually focus on events in your body: You have an incurable disease, your heart has weakened, your lungs are giving out. But the immediate effect is psychological. Gary Rodin, a palliative care specialist who was trained in both internal medicine and psychiatry, says this is the "first trauma"—the psychological and social effects of the disease.

The shock of confronting your own mortality can also happen at other times or in other ways, Coyle says: Maybe you look at yourself in the mirror and suddenly realize how skinny you are, or notice your clothes no longer fit well. Maybe you notice the way someone looks at you and recognize there's a change. "It's not necessarily verbal; it's not necessarily what other people are telling you," Coyle says. "Your body may be telling you, your soul may be telling you, or other people's eyes may be telling you."

WHY IS IT A CRISIS?

People are used to being vulnerable in normal existence—we know how to cope with that (most of us, most of the time). But that ability to cope falls sharply with the shock of finding out an illness is terminal. E. Mansell Pattison, one of the early psychiatrists to write about the emotions and responses of dying people, explains in *The Experience of Dying* why this realization marks a radical change in how people think about themselves:

> We anticipate a certain life-span within which we arrange our activities and plan our lives. And then abruptly we may be confronted with a crisis—*the crisis of knowledge of death*. Whether by illness or accident, our potential trajectory is suddenly changed.

People are able to create that sort of trajectory because we have a set of expectations and assumptions about life in general, a sense of the world that makes it possible for us to make it through the day, and plan for the future. These expectations are crucial for normal mental health, but they're based on a set of illusions that Lee says include the following: "overly positive beliefs about the self and expectations that there will always be tomorrow, that good people deserve good things happening to them, that it is possible to plan ahead into the future, and that the future looks bright." Most people don't examine these illusions until something deeply disturbing happens—something like being diagnosed with cancer. And when people learn they have a terminal disease, the illusions often come crashing down. "When cancer strikes, the belief system[s] that once provided a sense of stability, familiarity, and security are called into question."

WHAT DOES IT FEEL LIKE?

In a small 2011 Danish study, five patients with incurable esophageal cancer reported that after their diagnosis, their lives seemed to spin out of control. The patients wondered why *they* had received a fatal diagnosis. They asked, "Why me?" "Why now?" "What's going to happen?" "Am I going to die?" Some experienced despair and hopelessness; they felt their worlds were falling apart. They worried about the future, about their own grief. "I didn't care about anything," one patient said. "I had just about given up." Another said, "I felt like I was slipping into a depression. Even the simplest tasks were overwhelming. I couldn't handle the future."

Some people say they feel depression or despair or anger, or all three, Lee has found. They grieve. They grapple with a loss of meaning. A person's whole belief system may be called into question because dealing with treatment and the disease itself will affect almost every aspect of life.

During this crisis, a person's sense of anxiety can be close to intolerable. That's because patients are confronting a loss of identity and meaning. It makes sense that a person's first responses to a fatal diagnosis might include despair, anger, denial, meaninglessness, or depression.

But researchers also say the crisis is a phase that patients usually pass through—they can't remain long in this state of acute anxiety. Patients usually reach a peak of anxiety, which then subsides. In the 1970s, two Harvard researchers, Avery Weisman and J. William Worden, did a foundational study on existential plight, interviewing newly diagnosed cancer patients multiple times over the course of several months. After patients were diagnosed, the researchers found, they had significant, measurable changes in their emotional responses and understanding of the people and world around them. For almost all the patients in the study, existential concerns were the most important focuses in their lives, overriding concerns about any other consequences of their disease—physical symptoms, financial impacts, work, religion, or family.

The researchers also measured how long the existential plight lasted for patients diagnosed with a serious or life-threatening disease. They found that it usually began with the diagnosis and continued about two to three months, or approximately a hundred days.

In the beginning—soon after a diagnosis with a life-threatening disease—it's normal for patients to feel a high level of distress, Lee says. Like Weisman and Worden, she's found that that distress usually diminishes over the next three months.

Whenever uncertainty peaks and a dying person feels as if her life is threatened, her distress also increases. Those peaks tend to occur at the beginning of a diagnosis, at the start of treatment, such as chemotherapy, and at the start of surgery, for those patients who have it. Research has found that later peaks of anxiety and distress are not usually as severe as the first wave.

Researchers note that the crisis doesn't affect everyone in the same way. For some patients, the moment of recognition isn't deeply disturbing and it passes quickly. For others, finding out they have a serious or fatal disease reignites old emotional or social issues—unresolved grief from a divorce, or disappointment about not achieving one of their life dreams. Or they find that unrelated problems suddenly need new and different solutions and strategies: Strains in a relationship that were being ignored may need to be addressed directly through counseling, or finding a different place to live may have new requirements.

For many patients, the stunning recognition of their own mortality evaporates into denial for periods of time that can be jarring to family members or other observers.

THE REALIZATION THAT YOU'RE MORTAL MAY COME AND GO

"I don't know why I'm here—I'm not very sick," one patient at Mercy Hospice House, a residential hospice in Durango, Colorado, told me. "I think it's because my wife has the flu; maybe she needed a break." Another hospice patient kept saying he knew he'd whip his advanced cancer, just as he'd beaten other diseases or injuries in the past. He died a week later. Other patients sometimes chatter away blithely about plans to attend events or travel months or years in the future, as if there's no doubt they'll still be alive and able to participate.

Stephen, the man who lived for years knowing he had prostate cancer, never seemed to fully accept or understand that he had a fatal condition, even after the doctor told him his cancer had spread. "The existential slap? He didn't get it," says his wife, Jane. He may have had that deer-in-the-headlights moment in the doctor's office, but his existential crisis was brief and passed quickly. When a biopsy confirmed that the tumor was cancerous, Jane asked the doctor what he would do if he were in Stephen's place. He wouldn't waste his time seeking out costly further treatments that didn't really work, the doctor said. He encouraged Stephen to enjoy the time he had left with his family.

The conversation infuriated Stephen. He was a fighter and he'd wanted the doctor to suggest a potential miracle cure. He began searching for even more aggressive treatments. When his wife said she wouldn't take Stephen back to California to have his liver mapped—both the trip and the procedure seemed unnecessarily extreme and exhausting, she says—

Stephen had a friend drive him there. Later, after the disease had weakened him and he was spending most of his time in bed, friends would ask to visit. Stephen refused to see most of them. "They only want to come here because they think I'm dying," he told Jane.

When Stephen's symptoms required more help than Jane and part-time caregivers could provide, he finally enrolled in hospice. "You know what this means, to be on hospice?" Jane remembers asking him.

"Yeah, but I can get off anytime," he told her. A month or so later, he did leave hospice for two weeks so he could pursue curative treatments.

"I knew he was dying for a long time, and that's what was hard, I think," Jane says, because her husband still wouldn't acknowledge that fact. The weekend before Stephen died, a hospice nurse was at their home checking his vital signs. The nurse looked at him and said, "You know, you're in the dying process now." Jane remembers asking, "Are you hearing her?"

"Yes, I heard her," Stephen said. After the nurse left, Jane asked again, "Did you hear what she said?"

"That's just her opinion."

Another hospice patient with whom I spent four hours a week one memorable month certainly understood, somewhere in his mind, that he had a fatal brain tumor. When he'd undergone an initial brain surgery, his doctors told him the tumor would probably return. If it did, they said, there was nothing they could do to stop its growth. The tumor had indeed come back.

On our third visit, he asked why I was spending so much time with him. I told him I was there because I enjoyed our visits, but also because I was a hospice volunteer. I watched as he tried to assimilate the implications of being enrolled in hospice, although he'd certainly been informed before, multiple times by multiple people. Then he changed the subject. In our talks, his brain kept circling around the fact that his condition was fatal. When he discussed his tumor, he would say he was hoping for a miracle, in a tone that suggested he *expected* a miracle. And he would tell me his doctors *claimed* his tumor couldn't be cured, as if their medical opinions were suspect.

Even though this patient, like Stephen, spent most of his time in a state of denial, both probably had moments when they faced the truth. Stephen's wife recalls the few minutes in the doctor's office when he seemed to really grasp that he was dying, but the moment passed quickly. Palliative care doctors once believed patients were either in a state of denial or a state of acceptance. Now, Rodin and other researchers think people are more likely to move back and forth between those states. One researcher says a pendulum is a good metaphor for the way people face death, as they move back and forth between extremes of acceptance and denial. Weisman called this state "middle knowledge." He describes a patient who had accepted his own death, at least in the abstract. But when the patient experienced a period of stress, he began discussing future plans that would have been impossible because of his fatal disease. "Patients seem to know and want to know, yet they often talk as if they did not know and did not want to be reminded of what they have been told," Weisman writes. Some patients with a terminal disease seem to face an existential crisis, then return to a state of denial, and then double back to the crisis—perhaps more than once.

Weisman and Worden describe another case they say isn't unusual: A woman was told of her cancer diagnosis, only to report to interviewers that she didn't know what it was—and then make it clear she wasn't interested in receiving a diagnosis in the near future.

Still, it's almost impossible to maintain a steady sense of denial. The idea that you're dying doesn't stay at the forefront of consciousness, but once you've faced that fact, it remains somewhere in the background. Middle knowledge means that patients have *some* degree of awareness and insight about their condition, says Harvey Chochinov, a Canadian psychiatrist who specializes in palliative care. "They understand they have a relatively short life expectancy," he says, and yet there's a part of them that continues to need to maintain the status quo, and "the expectation is that there *is* a future."

Ideally, patients reach a perspective that allows them both to remain conscious of their condition and to participate fully in life. Rodin, the palliative care specialist and psychiatrist, explains it this way: "We think you sort of have to live with awareness of dying, and at the same time balance it against staying engaged in life . . . It's being able to hold that duality, which we call double awareness, which we think is a fundamental task."

CONFRONTING YOUR OWN MORTALITY ISN'T ALWAYS A CRISIS

The crisis of realization doesn't always entail mental suffering, and medical professionals who work with dying people say there are rare cases in which patients seem to skip this phase altogether, or at least experience it in a much less painful way. "People can gradually come to the realization," Coyle says. "No one *has* to go through the sudden shock of awareness."

Weisman and Worden note that some patients in their study never experienced the despair and depression of the existential slap. Many patients felt an impact but coped well and avoided the sense of "inevitable alarm and inexorable disaster."

Lee says researchers don't fully understand yet why some people don't search for meaning when they are given a fatal diagnosis. "Why me?" isn't a question everyone asks.

For some patients, maybe it's because they already knew they had a genetic predisposition, and having cancer fit into their expectations in life, she says. Or they've always believed they'd die young, or they've had close friends or family members who had cancer at a similar time in life. Somehow, the diagnosis fits their expectations, although researchers ultimately aren't sure why there are a few people who don't ask why cancer seems to have chosen *them,* as opposed to someone else.

Figuring out how to adapt to living with a life-threatening disease is usually a difficult but necessary cognitive process. If patients don't face the possibility of death and its consequences in their lives, they may become lost in depression and meaninglessness. But the patients who succeed often come to have a deeper appreciation of life and richer sense of who they are. Most patients do emerge on the other side of the existential crisis. And when they do, researchers have found that many discover new meaning.

YOU HAVE TO LIVE WITH THE RAIN

Jane says she doesn't know why her husband resisted his diagnosis so fiercely. One element was probably fear, she says. "But I think there's also personality types that are fighters: 'You tell me *this,* I'm going to do *that,*'" she says. "I think he had a little bit of that in him: 'Nobody's going to tell me when I'm going to die. I will say when that happens.'"

She says she's learned to try to avoid having expectations about how, and whether, people confront their own mortality: "At that point in life, nobody knows what we're going to think or say or do, so how can anybody else know, for somebody? You can't," she says. She says she really appreciates Stephen, a respectful, sweet man and loving husband. She even appreciates his persistence and strong will as he fought his disease when he might have been treasuring the last months with his wife and friends. "But it was hard for everybody else around him. It was hard on me. Because I knew he was leaving," she says.

Perhaps Stephen never really faced the fact that he was dying, or perhaps he was able to do that alone, when he was still conscious but could no longer speak. Jane yearned to have a healing conversation with him, one in which they talked about death and, through that difficult subject, discussed what was most important to them both in life. But since he was unwilling or unable to do so, she had that conversation on her own. She feels she was able to accept that Stephen was dying, that she was losing her husband. And through facing his mortality, she feels she's also been able to face her own.

When life is going well, it's easy to avoid difficult subjects, like a sense of meaninglessness, or the fact that everyone dies. But that's not easy to do when you're dying. "It's like trying to pretend you don't need an umbrella or something, or it's not raining, when it's pouring," Rodin says. "You can do that when it's drizzling, but eventually, you have to live with the rain."

chapter two
trajectories: patterns in how we die

IF YOU ASK PEOPLE how they'd *like* to die, the answers usually involve some form of "suddenly," and "unconsciously." In our sleep. Falling off a cliff. A quick accident of some kind. Imagine a graph representing the trajectory for sudden death: A straight horizontal line parallels the x-axis, until it intersects at right angles with a vertical line plunging straight down. This graph depicts a scenario in which someone enjoys a life of relatively good health, followed by a quick death without prolonged suffering. But of course, that's not the only way people die, or even the most common.

In a graph based on another trajectory, the horizontal line again parallels the x-axis at first, but then, rather than dropping straight down, falls at an angle like a slanted roof. After a life of good health, a patient's condition moves steadily down toward death. This is the trajectory many people think of in relation to terminal cancer.

In a third scenario, the horizontal line rises and dips in a series of small peaks and valleys as it gradually descends to the bottom. It's a picture of the way many patients with a serious chronic disease die as multiple complications bounce them in and out of the hospital. Each time, their recovery is a little less complete, until their systems finally fail.

A fourth graph described by Joanne Lynn, a physician and leading health care policy researcher, and her colleagues begins at a much lower point than the other three, and then very gradually sinks in a series of small dips. This graph illustrates long-term progressive frailty, caused by conditions like dementia, or a combination of serious illnesses. After years of slowly failing health, a person's condition continues to worsen until it reaches such a low level that something like the flu, pneumonia, or a broken bone may be the immediate cause of death.

This last scenario is the way most Americans will die. But the first two trajectories are still the deaths that many of us imagine for ourselves.

WE NEED NEW STORIES ABOUT DYING

Elderly nursing home patients used to tell Lynn they wanted to die like Cardinal Joseph Bernardin, who was diagnosed in the 1990s with pancreatic cancer. After the cancer spread to his liver, the Chicago church leader came to symbolize for many people a way to die with dignity. Bernardin spoke openly about his fatal condition and his fears associated with it, at the same time reaffirming his faith in God and the Catholic Church. "He said he was in too much pain to do any praying himself. And he was a very holy man; he was a very kind, gentle man, and he asked for others to pray for him," one hospice volunteer told me. "I'll always remember that." In Bernardin's last months of life, he added a ministry for people who had cancer or were dying of other causes, and he continued to attend to the needs of others until his last days.

His story, now mostly lost to younger generations, gave people at the time a way to imagine and talk about their upcoming deaths. Now, when people think about someone dying of a fatal disease, they still tend to imagine a particular scenario. "The story we know to tell is about the breast cancer patient who died at forty-five. Or the brain tumor patient," Lynn says. "We all know Brittany Maynard and her brain cancer, and we all know Teddy Kennedy and his, and Senator McCain." The particular illness or condition may differ, but these stories share a pattern: A life of good health is suddenly interrupted by a fatal diagnosis, followed by a steep decline and then a relatively rapid death. "Those are easy stories to tell, and they're sort of noble and they appeal to our heart strings," Lynn says. "Do we have any shared story of a person facing dementia?"

While a couple of recent movies have dealt with the subject, the popular understanding of how we die is only gradually starting to change. As baby boomers begin taking care of dying parents, for instance, the experience isn't what many had anticipated. Perhaps they expected to have a last few weeks to resolve old frictions with a dying parent, a time when the parent would say a few wise words or make grand pronouncements—only to discover their parents had dementia and the opportunity to talk was already past.

After observing their parents, people often begin to realize their own deaths won't match the scenarios they'd previously imagined.

It's not just dementia that lacks a shared cultural story; this is also true of any condition associated with a different dying pattern—conditions such as frailty, chronic pulmonary lung disease, heart disease, or even certain kinds of cancer. We're more likely to die from one of these conditions now, but we haven't had time to create new cultural stories.

DYING TRAJECTORIES

In their classic 1968 book, *Time for Dying,* sociologists Barney Glaser and Anselm Strauss sought to address that gap between the way we imagine death and the way it's more likely to transpire. As they studied medical professionals' expectations and the reality of individual deaths in hospitals, they also asked: How much control does a patient have over how her disease progresses, over how she dies? That depends at least in part, they concluded, on the kind of trajectory death takes, the pattern in how steadily or quickly a person approaches death.

Since Glaser and Strauss's study, other researchers, including Lynn, have built on the idea of dying trajectories. Lynn and her colleagues, for instance, set out to understand overall dying patterns so the health care system could do a better job of meeting the needs of the population as a whole. "We were saying that you probably could serve most people, most of the time, if you were really good at serving these . . . trajectories." And while the number and exact shapes of the trajectories differ, most trace the same general patterns.

THE SUDDEN DEATH TRAJECTORY

Sudden deaths are less common than other types of death in modern American life: Unintentional injuries are the third most likely cause of death. Heart attacks and strokes still kill people, but these can now often be treated with surgery or medications, which means they are less likely to lead to quick, unexpected deaths than they once were. Of course, people do still die from heart attacks or strokes. They die from traumatic injuries incurred in vehicle accidents or from falls. They die from drug overdoses or poison or accidental gunshot wounds. They are murdered or commit suicide.

The actual experience is necessarily brief.

The most common cause of sudden death worldwide is sudden cardiac death, often called a heart attack. But a heart attack can mean several different things. In one scenario, it can be the result of years of buildup of cholesterol in the heart arteries. Patients might have intermittent chest pains that worsen with exercise, followed by a heart attack, during which the patient is completely conscious, goes to the emergency room, and is treated. These heart attacks are not usually fatal for patients, most of whom are able to leave the hospital after just a few days, although some patients may later die of complications.

Another kind of heart attack is so serious that the blood supply to the heart muscle is suddenly blocked. Doctors call this *cardiac arrest secondary to acute myocardial infarction.* While patients may make a full recovery, they often do not. Patients who die from this condition are unlikely to suffer, or even know that they are dying. Most become unconscious because the heart blockage triggers ventricular fibrillation, when the heart's lower chambers stop beating in rhythm together, cutting off the supply of blood and oxygen to the brain.

This kind of death tends to be extremely rapid, and the people who experience it probably don't feel anything. Sudden cardiac death plunges its victims into almost instant unconsciousness; you simply can't continue to be conscious or alive for more than a second or two after your heart stops.

In contrast, people who have a major stroke may be very alert and awake. Strokes, which are caused by blockage of an artery to the brain, are almost always limited to one hemisphere. Patients don't die from the stroke itself, although its consequences often do lead to death. When they do, it's not typically a painful death: Stroke victims may have a headache, they may be confused or have trouble thinking of words, they may feel weak or have vision problems, but they don't usually experience much pain.

In addition to sudden cardiac deaths and strokes, emergency room physicians also see a range of fatal injuries that result in sudden deaths. The vast majority of these patients are either already unconscious, or they quickly sink into an unconscious state. When car accident injuries—the most common life-threatening traumas—are fatal, they almost always entail severe, traumatic brain injuries, which render victims immediately unconscious. It's unlikely that people even have time to become aware of what's going on—of any pain, or of the fact that they're dying.

There are rare traumatic accidents that are severe enough to cause death but that don't involve brain injuries. For instance, people who fall from great heights may break their pelvis, cutting tiny pelvic veins and bleeding out very quickly. The patient may go in and out of consciousness, but this is an extremely rare occurrence. Usually, anyone in an accident that's serious enough to kill them is likely to also suffer a brain injury that would lead instantly to unconsciousness.

If you received a fatal gunshot wound to the head, you'd also have no conscious experience of dying. But if you received a fatal gunshot wound that didn't affect your brain, you would be conscious and aware. You'd probably feel pain and psychological shock as you realized what was happening. But after a fairly short time, you would still lose consciousness as the level of oxygen in your brain plunged.

The most important thing for people to realize is that, at least in an emergency room, there is no reason for death to be a painful experience. Either it won't be painful because of the nature of the injury, or because of interventions by the medical team to alleviate your symptoms.

Often the reason sudden deaths in hospital emergency rooms are painless is "not because of anything we've done, but because that's just the physiological response to all these things—the final pathway: lack of oxygen, and then slipping into coma very quickly," says Jeremy Brown, director of the National Institutes of Health's emergency care office. "And in coma, by definition, you're not aware of your surroundings." For fatal traumatic injuries that happen in the field rather than in an emergency room, the case is sometimes different. For instance, if you were to break your neck in a fall from a horse, you might be conscious for a few seconds because your heart's still beating, but you'd be completely paralyzed from the neck down. And consciousness wouldn't last very long. Since you would no longer be breathing, you'd slip into a coma after about thirty seconds to a minute and then eventually die because your brain would not be getting enough oxygen. If people suffer a traumatic brain injury in the field, they will lose consciousness right away and therefore won't experience anything.

But in the rarer cases when people bleed to death, they may experience a sort of haziness in which they drift back and forth between consciousness and unconsciousness. However, even in those few moments of consciousness, it's unlikely they are aware of what's going on.

No matter what, if you were to die the kind of death represented by the first trajectory, it's unlikely your death would resemble those depicted on television or in the movies. Brown says, "I can't recall a case in which a patient had a severe injury"—severe enough to eventually prove fatal—"and that they were conscious to the point of understanding everything that was going on, and [then] sort of their eyes closed and they passed away as somebody might do on the battlefield in a movie, in the arms of a comrade. It may happen. But I've not experienced a single case like that."

Instead, it's the second trajectory that now most closely matches the fictional representations you'll read or see.

THE "CANCER TRAJECTORY"

After my mother discovered that her cancer was terminal, her life continued to be relatively normal for several years. She and my father entertained guests for dinner, traveled to visit friends and family and foreign places, and eventually packed up their belongings and moved to Colorado to be closer to me, my brother, and his family. After the move, my mother's series of chemotherapy treatments continued—as did her activities, such as bookkeeping for my father's business, serving on a local library board, and volunteering for hospice. She and my father took a daily walk with several neighbors, an entourage of dogs, and whatever family members could make it. They would hike partway up a nearby mountain, turning around at a small pile of rocks. After a while, they started adding a tiny rock to the pile every day—a talisman of good luck for my mother's health, maybe.

But in her last eight or ten months of life, my mother began to lose energy. She no longer made it to the cairn of rocks on their daily hikes. The walks kept shortening, until she only went the short distance to a place where the pavement stopped at the bottom of the hill. She stayed home more and entertained less. During a final trip to Australia with my father, she spent most of her time napping in hotel rooms or seeking out benches or chairs where she could read and rest. After they returned home, she was overcome with fatigue. A little over a month later, she died.

My mother's experience is a classic illustration of the second dying trajectory, in which a person's health remains relatively steady until the last five or six months of life, and then plunges rapidly.

Not all cancers follow this trajectory, but so many do that it's sometimes called the "cancer trajectory." Most patients with metastatic cancer can live relatively independent lives until their last few months; they can typically still walk, drive, and participate in activities—often for years after their diagnosis. Some patients become so accustomed to living with a fatal diagnosis that they're shocked all over again when they enter the steep decline—Durango palliative care doctor Anne Rossignol calls it "the cancer cliff"—and take to their beds, suddenly unable to lead active lives of engagement.

Because my mother's diagnosis was metastasized breast cancer, I asked Rossignol what she tells patients with this condition to expect when they're dying.

Every person is different, she says. But there are some very typical changes to your life: Your functional status will decline over time, so you won't be able to get around as well, she says. You usually lose your appetite. If a metastasized cancer spreads to your lungs and brain, which is not uncommon, you may start to have problems thinking. You might start having trouble with balance, depending on what part of the brain is affected. You might be short of breath and you might need oxygen at some point. And as your disease progresses, once you fall off the "cancer cliff," you may have more pain or other uncomfortable symptoms. You're likely to become less interactive with your family. Often, people will simply become very drowsy, go to bed and not get up again.

For patients whose disease follows this pattern, finding caregiving can be relatively easy, Lynn says. As in my mother's case, most cancer patients are "still very much nested in family and friends and community, and they're really, really sick for only a few months at most. And almost all families and communities can hold things together that long."

While it's difficult for doctors to know when the trajectory will take its sudden dive, once it does, they can estimate that patients will probably die within a few months. This fact makes the second trajectory a good fit for hospice, with its enrollment requirement that two doctors certify a patient is likely to die within six months. Indeed, for years, the majority of hospice patients in the United States had cancer, although that's no longer the case.

But even for many patients in this second trajectory, making an accurate six-month prognosis isn't easy. For patients whose dying progression follows the third or fourth trajectories, predicting the time of death can be still more difficult, or impossible. That means it's harder to make plans for what happens as you die, to take advantage of hospice benefits, or avoid disturbing trips to the intensive care unit. It can also be more difficult for you, your family, and even your doctor to face the fact that your condition is terminal.

NO ONE REALLY KNOWS WHERE THE STOP SIGN IN YOUR LIFE IS

About three years ago, I was assigned as a hospice volunteer to a new patient just before her hundredth birthday. When I walked into her home for the first time, her frail appearance was striking: She weighed a little over ninety pounds and her primary diagnosis was dementia. Occasionally, she had moments of lucidity, but she spent most of her time sleeping, hallucinating, or talking to people who were long dead. She had been enrolled in hospice because her doctors' best guess was that she would die within six months; if anyone had asked me at the time, I would have said she might die before my next visit the following week. But the patient, who has since "graduated" from hospice, was still alive at this writing.

No one wants to cause patients and their families the kind of turmoil and hardships that can result from inaccurate prognoses, and, when they can, most doctors avoid trying to predict exactly when someone will die. But hospice's six-month requirement can force their hands. Lynn believes the six-month prognosis is almost meaningless because there's not an agreed-upon statistical understanding of how to interpret it: Is the prediction based on an expectation that a scant majority—51 percent—of people with the prognosis will be dead within six months? Or is the expectation that 90 percent, or even 99 percent, will die within that period? "Anybody who's bet on the horses can understand that those are *very* different populations," Lynn says. "No one's been willing to deal with these issues, so not only do we not have the data, we have this sort of magical sense that a doctor knows where the stop sign is in your life course. Some people have a progressive and overwhelming illness that is on its own time frame." Estimating, even roughly, when you're going to die can be especially difficult for patients on the third dying trajectory.

THE "INTERMITTENT CALAMITY" OF ORGAN FAILURE TRAJECTORY

The third trajectory—the one that bounces up and down—is characteristic of heart failure and chronic obstructive pulmonary disease (COPD). Usually, patients feel reasonably good in their daily lives, until suddenly their condition worsens temporarily: "Most of the time, as you die of heart failure or respiratory failure, you're sort of in balance, and then some little thing happens: You eat a pretzel and tip yourself into heart failure. Or you've got a little bit of a cold, and you suddenly can't breathe well," Lynn explains. "So it's intermittent calamity. And sometimes you come back to where you were before, and sometimes, you've worn yourself out a little bit, and you come back not quite to where you were before."

One result is that patients on this trajectory are more likely to die in the ICU, receiving aggressive, last-minute treatments that are unnecessary and often don't match the patients' stated wishes. Marian Grant, the hospice and palliative care nurse practitioner, describes a patient who was admitted to the hospital seven times in six weeks for end-stage heart failure. "She kept calling 9-1-1, and then she'd come to the hospital, and they would fix her up a little bit, and then they'd send her home. A few days later she'd call, and she'd come back," says Grant, who is also a senior adviser at the Coalition to Transform Advanced Care. "It was crazy. But we didn't have another program to enroll her in. And she and her family didn't want hospice because they didn't think she was dying, which, of course, she was."

What does the dying process in this trajectory feel like? If you have congestive heart failure, your body's pump is failing. As it starts to work less and less well, you have more symptoms: You have difficulty breathing. You have fluid in your lungs and in your tissues. And if you don't have home hospice or palliative care, you're probably in and out of the hospital, even if you're doing everything right for the disease. The same is true for patients with chronic obstructive pulmonary disease—basically, lung disease: Your lungs are failing. You're more likely to get pneumonia or some other setback, which means you're also likely to check into a hospital more than once. With each hospital stay, your health tends to decline a little more, falling steadily downhill over time.

Doctors were once less likely to inform people that these conditions would ultimately prove fatal, Lynn says. Even when patients' health was so bad that they couldn't breathe in bed, the patients often thought their condition was just something they would live with, "and then something *really bad* happens to you." Patients believed they were waiting for a familiar fatal diagnosis such as cancer, although they actually already had a terminal condition. In the past fifteen to twenty years, medical professionals have become more likely to tell patients that their condition is probably terminal, and that information gives people choices, Lynn says. They might decide to forgo aggressive medical treatments, to make advance directives, and have important conversations with their families. People with heart or lung failure might have the chance to decide whether to use a ventilator or be given infusions or placed on a transplant list. Those kinds of aggressive treatments can often work for a long time, Lynn says: "I'm not saying that they're bad. It's just that it's a good thing people are now given the choice, in general, about whether to embark on them."

Still, many patients don't understand that they have a fatal condition. A 2015 study by a group of Scottish physicians interviewed patients in each trajectory to discover what it was like for them to live with a fatal condition. They found that patients on this third trajectory were often reluctant to face death, and, unlike their doctors and nurses, they might not even see their disease as terminal. Many just saw themselves as getting older.

That's also often true for people on the fourth dying trajectory: They simply don't know they're dying.

THE FRAILTY TRAJECTORY

"When is somebody dying? It's not even obvious anymore," says Rossignol, the Durango palliative care doctor. "We see these patients in the hospital and, are they dying? Are they not dying? Where are we in this process?"

When my mom was on hospice—she had COPD—she had a fall. She was a little, frail thing. She was ninety and broke her hip. Was it the dog she tripped on? Was it her oxygen? It didn't matter. What mattered was that she fell.

Now I didn't say, "You're going to die because of this fall, Mom." I knew that was going to happen, but that's not how my mom could absorb things. She couldn't absorb what this was going to look like. That's not how she lived her life. My mom, with eight kids, the way she could manage was keeping things in different buckets. All I could say was, "Mom, we're not going to fix it. We're in quite a pickle here because you're not strong enough to do surgery." She could hear that. "We're in quite a pickle. I'm not going to let you hurt. We're going to keep you home. We're going to take care of you and we'll all be here." She could hear that. She knew she was dying. I didn't have to say, "Mom, you're dying." Because that didn't fit my mom. Everybody's so different, so when you approach people, for me, anyway—some people are just super-intuitive; they're just so good. And some people aren't.—MICHELLE APPENZELLER, CLINICAL DIRECTOR AT HOSPICE OF MERCY IN DURANGO

The condition that the majority of people in the United States will probably die of doesn't even have a name widely recognized as a cause of death: After years with an increasing number of chronic diseases, weakened by aging, many people will become frail, a condition "where we are in a very fragile balance with our environment for a very long time," Lynn explains. "And we are essentially waiting for some little thing to overwhelm us because we have very little resilience—or, for the body to finally, really give out, after a very long course." Many doctors still don't recognize that frailty is a syndrome, Lynn says. Furthermore, because it's not typically listed on death certificates, frailty isn't included in the Centers for Disease Control and Prevention's list of leading causes of death. As it sometimes is with organ failure, the immediate cause of death may be something that wouldn't ordinarily be fatal, such as a small heart attack or small stroke, or even a cold: "And that's how most of us will die," says Lynn. "We'll succumb to the complications of something really trivial—and the doctor won't even put it on the death certificate—what are you going to say, 'died of a cold'?"

One reason so many people die of frailty is that more and more people are living longer and surviving with multiple chronic conditions: "By 2025, the percentage of people aged 65 years and over will be almost 30% in developed and almost 15% in less developed regions [worldwide]," psychiatrist and researcher Joao Solano and his colleagues point out. "While this increase in longevity is welcome, as a consequence more and more people are dying from chronic, rather than acute, diseases. They will usually have endured several symptom complexes for many years."

In a blog post, Lynn describes what dying of frailty looks like in her ninety-six-year-old mother's case: "losing nearly half of her weight, barely able to get up from a chair, having a plethora of symptoms with no treatable etiology, and yet having enough heart, lungs, kidney, and liver functions to go on for a while." Like Lynn's mother, a majority of people in the United States can now expect to depend on someone else for daily care and support in their last two years of life. *Two years.* Someone dying from dementia might need daily care for eight or ten years, past the point when family and friends are worn out. These patients need much more personal care, such as being bathed, dressed, or spoon-fed, and for much longer, than patients in other dying trajectories typically do.

The health care system isn't set up for people who die of frailty or dementia or other conditions in this fourth trajectory, Lynn says, but she believes that will change. "I think we will gradually get there, but it would matter to get there more quickly, because we're making a big mistake. We're inflicting suffering on patients and families in a way that we probably didn't really want to do, because we never learned to do anything else."

Lynn and her fellow researchers developed their set of dying trajectories in the hopes they could help prevent that suffering. They believed the trajectories would aid health care policy makers in planning for different kinds of deaths. But the dying trajectories can also help individual patients pull back and see the big picture: What clues are there about whether you've started down that pathway or not? About what your remaining days or months might be like?

Of course, while trajectories provide some sense of perspective, one of the key hints about what dying may be like is your specific condition.

HOW MUCH DOES YOUR PARTICULAR DISEASE AFFECT HOW YOU DIE?

Every year, the CDC issues an updated list of the ten most common causes of death in the United States. Here's the most recent list, published in 2018 but based on 2016 numbers, starting with the most common cause:

1. Heart disease
2. Cancer
3. Unintentional injuries
4. Chronic lower respiratory disease (COPD, emphysema, bronchitis, asthma, etc.)
5. Stroke
6. Alzheimer's disease
7. Diabetes
8. Influenza and pneumonia
9. Kidney disease
10. Suicide

This isn't the only way the CDC breaks down its data, and when you examine the causes of death more closely, the stark certainty of the list begins to waver. For instance, the organization also produces a chart of the top causes of death divided by age group. If you're between 45 and 64 years old, the top two leading causes of death are reversed. If you die when you're between the ages of 15 and 34, the cause is much more likely to be violent: Suicide is the second leading cause of death for this group, followed by homicide. If you're between the ages of 1 and 44, the leading cause of death is unintentional injury. And of course, it's not just your age that affects how you're most likely to die. The CDC also provides charts based on socioeconomic status, race, and where you live.

By the time you die, the leading causes of death will almost certainly have shifted. Who knew in the 1970s that AIDS would take such a toll on the lives of young people in the United States in the 1990s? And how many Americans had even heard of the Zika virus until recently? Other serious diseases that were once rare could sweep the country. At the same time, new treatments and lifestyle changes could continue to reduce fatalities from the diseases that now top the CDC's list. From 2015 to 2016, death rates increased in three categories—unintentional injuries, Alzheimer's, and suicide—but decreased for all the other top ten causes of death. After effective treatments were developed, the percentage of Americans who die from AIDS has dropped substantially. Rates of heart disease and cancer are also declining, most likely because of new treatments and because significantly fewer Americans smoke than we once did.

But we all have to die of *something*. So "to prevent one way of dying is, in effect, to 'create' another," notes James Hallenbeck in his book, *Palliative Care Perspectives*. Whenever the medical profession finds effective treatments or preventions for a particular cause of death, there's a corresponding increase in deaths from other causes: "Even very good things like seatbelts are 'carcinogenic' in that by decreasing the chance of dying in car accidents, seatbelts proportionately increase the probability of growing older and dying from other diseases such as cancer," he writes.

In early 2018, five patients were staying at a hospice residence I visited. One had a diagnosis of pancreatic cancer; another had mesothelioma, a rare form of cancer; and a third had ALS, also known as Lou Gehrig's disease. A fourth patient had prostate cancer, and the fifth had gastrointestinal hemorrhaging. Each was struggling with different symptoms, and each person's ability to do normal, everyday activities had been affected in different ways. N, the patient who had gastrointestinal hemorrhaging, had been confined to her bed for weeks. When she first arrived at the hospice residence, she was eager for company. She chatted happily with volunteers and staff members about crocheting a quilt, and about returning home to see her dog and spend the night. A few weeks later, she was spending most of her time sleeping, and she needed assistance just to walk to the bathroom.

D, the ALS patient, couldn't move his arms and hands by himself because of nerve damage, so he needed help eating and drinking, or just checking his e-mail or changing a television channel. In a room down the hall, T, the patient with pancreatic cancer, still went out to lunch with a friend who pushed him in his wheelchair to a nearby restaurant. But he also suffered from bouts of severe pain, while N said she had no pain, and she wasn't taking medications for any symptoms. How many of these patients' symptoms and impacted abilities were caused by their particular condition, and how many depended on the stage of the disease or other factors?

Solano and his colleagues compared cancer patients' symptoms with those of patients who had heart disease, AIDS, chronic obstructive pulmonary disease, or renal disease. They found some differences in symptoms based on which disease a patient had: Patients diagnosed with heart disease or chronic obstructive pulmonary disease were much more likely to need help dealing with breathlessness. AIDS patients were more likely to have problems with nausea, insomnia, and diarrhea, while cancer patients were more likely to have anorexia. But the researchers also found that a core group of symptoms affected patients with all five of the conditions they studied. More than 50 percent of patients with any of the conditions studied experienced pain, fatigue, and breathlessness. "There seems to be a common pathway that people with far advanced progressive diseases have to face," the researchers conclude.

When Karen Steinhauser and her coauthors did a study comparing patients with three different serious diseases, they subtitled it, "Does Diagnosis Matter or Is Sick, Sick?" Their conclusion seems to be both yes and no. Where patients lived, how severe the disease was, and the patients' emotional and social well-being were more important than the actual disease in determining their experiences, the researchers write. The particular diagnoses had less significant effects on patients' quality of life.

Still, the diseases did matter. A year or more before they died, patients who had cancer could function better than those with chronic heart failure or chronic obstructive pulmonary disease. The researchers found that the situation reverses in the last few months of life, when patients with cancer have less ability to function independently than patients with heart or lung disease.

Joan Teno, a University of Washington professor whose research focuses on end-of-life care and policy issues, came to a similar conclusion when she and her coauthors analyzed how much patients' ability to participate in daily activities declined, depending on their fatal disease. Patients dying of non-cancer conditions, such as heart failure, COPD, or diabetes, had more difficulty in performing daily activities a year before they died than those with cancer, according to their study. But close to death, cancer patients had the hardest time with these activities. About 14 percent of cancer patients in the study had trouble getting up out of bed or out of a chair a year before their deaths, compared to 35 percent of the patients in the non-cancer group. But in the last five months of life, 63 percent of cancer patients struggled to get out of bed, while 50 percent of non-cancer patients shared this difficulty.

Ultimately, although people die of many different causes, there are only a few routes to death—Marian Grant estimates maybe twenty or thirty. And no matter the disease or patterns, the final months of life for people with a fatal disease share many commonalities.

TIMING IS EVERYTHING

When Lynn and her coauthors began their study that resulted in the dying trajectory analysis, they wanted to improve health care for dying people by thinking more like a business: "If you were at the board table for Marriott Hotel, you would be thinking in terms of what are the populations that might use our motels and hotels, and you would build somewhat different environments for a business location, or a resort location, or a location at an intersection of interstates," Lynn explains. "You'd be thinking in terms of, what is it people need in different situations?"

But the researchers soon realized that *time* played a more important role than the type of fatal condition a patient might have. Depending on the length of time that patients had difficulty functioning independently, their needs might be very different. For instance, someone who dies relatively quickly, following the first or second trajectory, needs caregiving for a much shorter amount of time than someone whose dying process lasts longer. And a person who has advanced dementia for years is more likely to need support for staying engaged in meaningful activities as long as possible. He might need help bathing, dressing, and eating.

What patients themselves are discovering is that the length of time between being diagnosed with a fatal disease and dying has grown. Because of the treatments and technologies of modern medicine, we seem to have created a larger liminal space where people linger between life and death for longer and longer periods—a time when they know they have a terminal disease but are still very much alive. That existential slap of knowledge changes you permanently. But are you *dying*, simply because you know you have a terminal condition? Or are you now living in a new place, somewhere between life and death?

chapter three

after the diagnosis: in the land of living/dying

AFTER MY MOTHER received her diagnosis of stage 4 breast cancer, and after she had braved radiation, chemotherapy, and a double mastectomy, she and my father went for one last checkup with Brenda, my mother's personable oncologist at Vanderbilt University Medical Center. It was a friendly visit, the three of them chatting away about my mother's wonderful progress and apparent health in the year since her last treatment, about my parents' plans to move to Colorado, about Brenda's own upcoming move to a different cancer center.

They were already saying their good-byes when Brenda remembered she hadn't checked the results of my mother's scan. She popped out of the examination room, promising to return quickly. When she did, her expression had turned grim: My mother's cancer was not just growing but had spread to her liver. "My liver spots looked like the hide of a hyena," my mother would later write.

Neither Brenda nor anyone else could tell her how much longer she had to live. While chemotherapy treatments could check the cancer's growth or even reduce the number and size of her tumors, my mother now realized the disease was going to kill her. She was not alone in this strange and indefinite predicament: Hundreds of thousands of Americans live with a fatal diagnosis. In an article about the experiences of patients with advanced cancer, palliative care specialists Gary Rodin, Rinat Nissim, Sarah Hales, and their colleagues call it "the land of the living/dying." Patients in their study describe this state as "an unnatural place in which to live, first and foremost, because it involves a new relationship with one's personal finitude."

The patients all saw death itself as an expected, natural part of life; it was the liminal state that felt artificial and foreign: "What they found unnatural about the land of the living/ dying is the continual knowing, as one participant put it, that one is 'always on the verge of dying,'" the researchers explain. "To live with this constant knowing was a strange and almost indescribable experience, far from the familiar range of their experience and the experiences of those around them."

My mother would survive another four and a half years with the knowledge of her fatal diagnosis. If you had asked any of us—my mother or father, the rest of our family, their friends—at the time, I don't think we could have predicted what those four and a half years would entail. We didn't anticipate the frustrations and difficulties. We didn't foresee that we still had so many experiences left to share with her— activities like bicycling in Holland or hiking in the mountains or sharing family brunches. We didn't expect the richness of that time, or the delight.

AFTER THE INITIAL DIAGNOSIS, THEN WHAT?

The cultural expectation sometimes seems to suggest there are only two categories of human life, writes Joanne Lynn, the hospice physician and policy adviser: Either you're semi-immortal, or you're breathing your last gasp.

One hears people say, "He's not dying yet," of a person living with fatal lung cancer. Generally, that means he's not yet taking to bed, losing weight, and suffering from pain, as would be expected when dying is all that he can do. But the category is used as if one is either "temporarily immortal"—which is the usual state of human beings—or "dying," in which case the person is of a different sort, having different obligations and relationships.

If you're dying, you're supposed to be pretty much finished with life, but that's not true for most, Lynn writes. People diagnosed with a terminal disease know—at least on some level—that their condition will eventually kill them. But they also have so much living ahead of them.

"We are not half dead people who cannot do anything," says a patient quoted in a study by the Canadian hospice pioneer Balfour Mount and his colleagues.

Ever since the widespread popularity—and frequent misunderstanding—of Elisabeth Kübler-Ross's five stages of grief, scholars have been wary about dividing people's dying process into stages. Kübler-Ross's work was groundbreaking, bringing public attention to the plight of people who lay dying in hospitals that couldn't admit they *had* dying patients. She also offered the American public a way to talk more openly about death and dying, a skill many seem to have forgotten as the dying were moved out of homes and into hospitals beginning around the middle of the nineteenth century. But Kübler-Ross's five stages have been read as prescriptive, rather than descriptive—as a sort of list of steps any grieving person must pass through in order to "do" grief correctly: First, you need to experience denial, then anger, then bargaining, then grief and depression, and, finally, acceptance.

That's not how people work. Reactions to grief don't arise in a particular order. And experiencing one of them—say, denial—once, doesn't mean you won't experience it again.

Perhaps you initially deny the fact that your illness can't be cured, then accept it, and then deny it again and again. Or you may skip stages entirely, or you might experience additional emotions that Kübler-Ross never described.

I did not go through the five stages of grief (not being religious, with whom would I bargain or be angry?). For me, it was just an unwavering sense of "this sucks," but there have been rays of light. In those early days, feeling sick before chemotherapy began and worse after, I would have preferred to have died in a car crash on the way to the scanner. But on further reflection, wasn't it better to have been allowed to come back for a while to say good-bye, to spend time with loved ones and exchange kind words with friends, colleagues, and trainees in public, in private, and in e-mail?—FRANK LEDERLE

Although misinterpretations of Kübler-Ross's five stages skewed the picture of what patients actually experienced, research does support the idea that the process of dying might be broken into different parts, each of which has a different feel. In *The Experience of Dying,* E. Mansell Pattison divides dying into three main phases: the acute crisis phase, the chronic living-dying phase, and the terminal phase. After the initial shock of discovering that they have a fatal disease—the acute crisis, or the existential slap—most people enter a sort of middle phase that lasts from the time of diagnosis until the last few days of their lives. Pattison calls it the *living-dying interval.* While Pattison's name for the phase emphasizes time, Rodin and his colleagues' label—*the land of living/dying*—highlights place. Both names suggest that in this phase, the normal measurements of living simply don't apply. The state can feel like something outside ordinary time and space.

Most of us can now expect to experience this long period of

dying, a period in which we live for weeks, months, or even years with the knowledge that we have a fatal disease.

WHAT'S NEW IN THE LAND OF LIVING/DYING?

It can feel as if technology and medical progress have made the living/dying interval longer lasting and much more widespread in modern Western cultures than it was, say, a hundred years ago. David Jones, a professor of the culture of medicine at Harvard University, says it's nearly impossible to know for sure—the stories that have survived are by and about the people who had money and education, not the vast majority of people living at the time.

But we do know that lingering terminal diseases are nothing new. In Thomas Mann's classic novel, *The Magic Mountain,* tuberculosis patients spend months or years at a Swiss sanatorium in the Alps. They have come there hoping for a cure, although most will eventually die of their disease. Time flows, or stops, or eddies out, and life is lived in a state of limbo, a space between life and death. The patients in Mann's book were fictional, but their years of living with a disease they suspected or knew was terminal were not. A chart in the first issue of *The New England Journal of Medicine* in 1812 lists the leading causes of death at the time, and consumption—tuberculosis—led other causes by a significant margin.

Although it's hard to be certain whether the percentage of people with lingering terminal illnesses has increased significantly, Jones says, the patients who fall into that category might well feel sicker than dying people did a hundred years ago. For example: "The whole category of people with chronic renal failure on dialysis—those people would have died of dropsy over months, ages ago," he says. "Now we keep them alive for years on dialysis. And for that category of patients, there's a mode of survival, but it's an uncomfortable mode of surviving that wouldn't have existed previously."

Still, the modern land of living/dying is very different from that of people a hundred years ago. In the nineteenth century, almost all dying people would have continued to live at home, under the care of their family members. Many would never have visited a doctor at all, Jones points out. The treatments for terminal diseases have also changed, and the effects of these sometimes have serious impact on the lives of patients. Nineteenth-century treatments for fatal diseases could be painful, but nothing then equaled the side effects of certain kinds of modern chemotherapy. "Essentially, people who have been through bone marrow transplants are brought to the brink of death by the treatment, in hopes of bringing them back. And certainly, many cancer patients, especially ones who are actively fighting until the end, are chronically sick not just from the disease but also from the treatment's side effects," Jones says.

"So I think there probably is a category of cancer patients who are deathly ill for a long period of time from the combined effects of chemo and cancer, who are sicker for longer, because they can keep really sick people alive in a way they couldn't have in the past."

WHAT THE LIVING/DYING INTERVAL FEELS LIKE

He used to do laps around the furniture—I think the highest he ever got to was twenty-five laps. He'd wear his Fitbit. He was working up to where he could go out on the sidewalk down at the park. One of the nurses and I took him down there. I had a really great walker for him; it wasn't wobbly at all. We had also taken his wheelchair; we had to use that to get him back to the car. That was his last outing, and he died a week later.

*And it's almost like that was his peak day—he got to do
that—but his body just couldn't keep doing it.
I would ask him sometimes, "So, what's holding you
here? What is it?"
And he would just kind of sit there, and he'd go,
"Well, it's the dogs, and you, and the birds."
In January of last year, he said, "I just want to be
here so I can watch the migratory birds come through,"
because we get tons of western tanagers here and it's
really fun. And I said, "Okay," and I put out the suet,
and we watched, and they were beautiful. Then after
they left, the woodpeckers were out there, and the
other kinds of birds that came later . . . I think he kept
thinking, "Oh, I'll last six more months." I think he
really thought that. But a few years ago, he said, "You
don't ever have to worry about taking care of me because
if I can't hike anymore, I'm out of here." The way we see
death changes.* —WIDOW OF A CANCER PATIENT

The first hospice patient I worked with as a volunteer
lived in a local nursing home where her husband, in his early
nineties, came to visit every day and stayed from breakfast
until after dinner. They struggled at first with the institutional bureaucracy that made it difficult for her to accomplish
straightforward goals: a reasonably short time waiting on
the toilet for an aide's help, meals that tasted good, timely
hair appointments—and help getting outside once in a while
to smoke a cigarette. But the couple eventually charmed the
nursing home staff and other residents. After a month or so,
they established a routine. In almost any weather, the husband
would wheel his wife outside to eat her meals, sometimes even
when the patio tables were encrusted with ice. Other residents
would drop by, rolling up in a wheelchair or scooting over from
a nearby table. The husband would tell stories about his fam-

ily's travels across the West, back when he and his wife were working ranches as a cooking team, or the story of when he and his wife first met as teenagers. She would roll her eyes or laugh, pecking at her meal and enjoying a cigarette before returning to the oxygen tank in her room. Twice, when we were alone, she complained about frustrations with her husband or her life at the nursing home. But overall, she seemed to have reached a place of relative contentment as she waited to die. It would be more than a year before that happened.

When scholars study the mental states of dying patients, they often survey family members or doctors or nurses—for understandable reasons. But witnesses tend to describe a lower quality of life for dying people than patients themselves do.

When researchers actually talk to dying people, they discover something different. In 2016, a group of Spanish nurses published an analysis of thirteen studies, each of which was based on interviews with advanced cancer patients. Three common themes emerged from those conversations: Patients described living with their cancer as a unique process in which their chief goal was to live as normally as possible. They said their support networks, especially their relationships with relatives or close friends, were crucial to them. And they said their interactions with the health care system—elements such as the quality of their hospital experiences or their access to the kind of specialty health care they needed—were critical.

In other studies, patients with lingering terminal diseases say they feel a loss of control over their lives. More than anything else, they seek to live as normally as possible. They say they sometimes feel better when their lab reports indicate they should feel worse—and vice versa. They say their relationships with other people have changed in important ways. They struggle with increasing dependence on others, and with physical pain and physical changes.

But they are not necessarily unhappy.

Researchers have begun to measure positive as well as negative mental states in dying people. Studies have found that people with serious disabilities or life-threatening illnesses often rate their quality of life just as highly as the general population does—or, in at least one study, the seriously ill people may rate life quality even more highly. A 2005 study of people with advanced amyotrophic lateral sclerosis—Lou Gehrig's disease—reported that few of the patients were depressed, and none of them became more depressed as death approached. A 2000 study about the last six months of life for patients with congestive heart failure found that even though difficult physical symptoms grew worse close to death, the perceived quality of life didn't decline significantly for most of the patients.

People who are diagnosed with terminal diseases describe parts of their experience as both mentally and physically painful, and depression and anxiety are common. But they often say their terminal illnesses lead to positive experiences they never would have had otherwise. And their psychological and existential states have been shown to improve right up until a few days before they die.

Most people diagnosed with a fatal condition experience shifts in how they think about their impending deaths. The distress and anxiety brought on by that first existential slap usually diminish or go away, but the stress of having a fatal disease still waxes and wanes. Some patients describe the changing states of emotions they experience as being like waves.

Two doctors in Israel, Craig Blinderman and Nathan Cherny, interviewed a group of forty patients with advanced cancer after they had passed the acute phase of their initial diagnosis. What the researchers discovered is revealing: First of all, they found that death and dying weren't their patients' most important concerns. After confronting their initial diagnosis, about 50 percent said they didn't think about death and dying. Several patients who said they *were* contemplating their own deaths also said they'd developed coping methods and didn't find the thoughts about death distressing. Many reported they felt they were dealing well with issues such as loss of dignity or meaning, and guilt or disappointments about the past.

Dying people don't necessarily consider themselves sick: One study found that "one-third of a sample of fifty cancer patients with active disease considered themselves to be 'fairly healthy' and two-thirds reported being 'very healthy,' including twelve who died during the study." Ideally, Rodin says, patients strike a balance, both facing their impending deaths and living as fully as they can in the time they still have remaining: "You need to be able to face the end, face the fact that life is coming to an end and make plans and so on, and also manage your cancer," he says. Patients usually need to work on end-of-life practicalities: organizing financial matters, writing or updating wills, making funeral or memorial plans. Their lives may also grow busy with doctors' appointments and medical treatments. But patients need to save energy for relationships, meaningful activities, contemplation—for *life*—at the same time, Rodin cautions. "And people who can't think about their cancer and dying and all those things, can't plan, and also come down with a crash. And people who are swallowed up by it, who think about it all the time . . . have already given up on life." He and his colleagues say patients need to do both; they need to maintain a double awareness.

PEOPLE WORK HARD IN THE LAND OF LIVING/DYING

In a time when people were much more likely to spend their dying days—or weeks, or months—in the hospital, Nessa Coyle was a nurse in a ward where most of the patients had terminal diseases. She began to notice how much information those patients were trying to absorb, and how many different experts and staff members they often interacted with. At the end of the day, she says, "we'd see them sort of sitting in bed in silence, and not saying very much, and taking in a lot of information . . . from many, many people from different medical specialties . . . giving them information, perhaps in a different way, both verbally and nonverbally."

Coyle started making time to sit down with patients to see if she might discover what they were thinking and feeling. In those conversations, she was struck by the fact that patients in the advanced stages of disease were *working*—hard. They were trying to plan for how their illnesses might affect their jobs and home lives. They were trying to protect family members, to plan for providing for family, and to adapt to their own changing family roles. They were making complicated decisions about their medical care: "There's a lot of work going on as they're absorbing the information from these different sources that they're getting each day," Coyle says. And she notes that patients had to be mentally alert to nuances in communication because the information they were gathering nonverbally—from people's expressions, tones of voice, doctors' and nurses' actions—sometimes contradicted what people said. "They also learn that words have meaning, and if you say certain things, it may affect the sort of care that you get," Coyle says. Patients learned that if they complained of a lot of pain, their chemotherapy treatments—treatments that might have the potential to lengthen or save their lives—could be placed on hold until the pain was under control.

Coyle eventually decided to conduct a small study of people in the advanced stages of disease. She interviewed seven patients multiple times about how their conditions affected their attitudes about life and death: "They struggled with fear for their lives, multiple symptoms, urgent treatment decisions, and changing relations to self, family, and place in the world," she writes. Just when these patients were at one of the most vulnerable points in their lives, their burdens of work had increased: "This unfamiliar work was visited upon individuals who were sick, weakened, and vulnerable and who now struggled to survive."

And one of the largest drains on patients' time and energy, Coyle learned, was trying to regain a sense of control.

LOSING CONTROL

What's different about patients with a terminal illness is that they have a pretty good idea of what will kill them—although they, like any of us, could also die in an unexpected car crash or unforeseen accident. They also have a better idea than most people of the times of their deaths: soon.

But dying people are still caught in a paradox. They know they will die in the near future, but they don't know exactly when, and that period of doubt could stretch from weeks to months, or even to years. One of the most difficult feelings dying people say they experience is caused by uncertainty. "It's like a time bomb in your stomach," says a patient quoted in one study. "You know there's a tumor sitting there, and at will or at whim, you know, it will choose to activate."

In the study by Rodin and his colleagues of people with advanced cancer, that uncertainty was one thread in a general feeling of losing control: Patients didn't know how rapidly their diseases might progress or affect what they could do. That, in turn, meant they didn't know whether they could continue working or engaging in the activities they cared about. They didn't know whether or when they might lose the ability to travel or walk or live independently, or when they might lose control of their kidneys and bowels.

After one of my friends was diagnosed with terminal cancer, she maintained her athletic outdoor life. She rafted the Grand Canyon, skied in the backcountry, and continued to mountain-bike and hike—all in the last year or so before she died. When the cancer began a rapid progression in her last couple of months of life, she and her husband were caught off guard. In their case, the suddenness of her transformation from active athleticism to active dying was surprising and unsettling.

The hospice patients and their families I've witnessed have sometimes experienced the same unexpected jolt. The patients know they have a fatal disease, but they are startled and upset when they start declining rapidly. They expected this change, patients or family members will say, but later— maybe after a few more months, another year.

Patients in Rodin's study were more frustrated by uncertainty itself than by the thought of dying. As a result, the goal they mentioned most frequently was controlling the dying process in some way. They tried to accomplish this by treating their diseases as aggressively as possible, and also by toying with the idea of ending their own lives, although none of them actually attempted suicide. Even when chemotherapy treatments resulted in substantial side effects and provided few benefits, patients would continue the treatments for months. While the patients sometimes saw the chemotherapy treatments as life-saving, there was another motive at play: "This tendency reflected not only their desire to prolong living but also their fear of an uncontrollable dying process," the researchers explain.

Ultimately, the treatments provided only a partial sense of control, as one patient reported: "It's like super gambling because you don't know what's going to happen and nobody knows what's going to happen. One bad reaction and—bang! You are out [dead]."

This attempt to regain control by pursuing aggressive treatments sometimes made patients' interactions with the health care system overwhelming, Rodin and his coauthors note: "The tactic of maximizing treatment options demands considerable time and energy, constituting a 'full-time job,' as several participants put it." The chemotherapy treatments themselves make people weak, and they often have difficult side effects. Negotiating more clinics and medical professionals and providers also requires significant effort. Half the patients in the study obtained a second opinion about treatments, and patients often went to still another set of doctors to deal with the side effects of chemotherapy. Especially for patients who had dependent children or needed to work to support themselves and their families, managing their illness and seeking to maximize their treatments put their lives in a sort of overdrive.

Another way patients sometimes tried to regain control of their lives was by trying to figure out the cause of their advanced disease. They tried to establish who was at fault. One patient hypothesized that if stress had caused his disease, then reducing stress might also act as a cure: "There is nothing concrete about stress causing lymphoma but it is in the right system—the lymphoid system and neuroendocrine hormones. My mind permitted me to get lymphoma and my mind could cure lymphoma. I had to change my lifestyle."

Another patient, discussing whether the medical system had somehow caused or contributed to her fatal disease, put it this way: "I blame them, I blame myself, it's all a mess but the fact that I may die soon is somebody's fault."

YOUR RELATIONSHIPS WITH OTHER PEOPLE CHANGE

When you know you're going to die, you're not the only one affected—and your family and friends can prove to be sources of both support and friction. One woman in a study of patients with ovarian cancer told researchers that her disease had both brought her closer to her husband and increased the stress on their relationship:

We didn't fight for a long time after my diagnosis
because who cares if you'd pick up your clothes off the
floor . . . because we are just in love and we have each
other, and we don't know how long that will last and
that kind of stuff. And we go from that to under so
much stress because of it and feeling so much fear that
we're at each other's throats. You know, just feeling
really, really stressed out about stuff.

Studies show that a patient's family typically becomes more
important after an illness has been diagnosed. People realize
their time together is finite, and they often want to spend less
time on lower priorities and more time with each other.

Friends and acquaintances may also play a more central
role in patients' lives than they have previously, but a lot depends on their responses to the disease. Patients say they feel
other people often treat terminally ill people differently. One
woman told researchers her disease had "made me aware of
how uncomfortable people are around cancer patients. And
it's been challenging just to . . . sort of try to break through
that with people you know . . . it's amazing the people that you
know . . . almost try to avoid you." But the same study finds
that patients also say people they didn't expect to do so step
forward. One woman said her ovarian cancer had "kind of cut
off some relationships and made others much stronger":

There are some friends with whom I have no contact.
Some people are just totally unable to handle it. And
it was very upsetting but understandable . . . Other
people, other acquaintances will say, "I am taking you
on such and such a day and no two ways about it."

At least one study has found that cancer patients receive
more social support from family, friends and caregivers than

healthy people do. And the worse the patients' conditions were, the more support they received.

One of the greatest concerns patients report about their relationships is a fear of a growing dependence on others. Patients say they worry about becoming a burden, about others having to take care of their basic physical needs, and about not being able to fulfill their usual roles within the family.

Roles do shift. Patients who have been the breadwinners or run a household lose that ability as they weaken, and they find themselves needing to be cared for. And while caregivers often welcome the burden of taking care of someone they love, that doesn't mean it isn't stressful for them, as well as for the patient. But Ira Byock, a physician who has written extensively about dying, argues that even if dying people do become a burden, their families and friends benefit from the very act of rallying to their aid: "Allowing others to support and care for us when we're ill is also essential to the well-being of our communities. Indeed, refusing to be cared for erodes the living bonds that form a community."

In his clinical work, Byock says he'd often meet people who were struggling with the fear of being a burden. That was true of his own dying father, who told Byock, "It's so messy . . . just take me to the hospital. They'll take care of me."

Byock says he told his father he was willing to do that: "We could take you to the hospital and pump you up with antibiotics and then get you back to New Jersey," he remembers telling him. "I'd travel with you on the plane; I'm pretty sure you'd make it there, and then, you know, we could put you in the hospital there, and you could die in the hospital."

But Byock told his father he'd prefer to care for him at home. "And he looked at me, and then he looked away from me, kind of straight ahead beyond the foot of his bed. And then, without looking back at me, he just nodded his head a couple of times."

Byock believes his father agreed to stay at home because he

realized that was what his family wanted most. "He figured out that we needed to care for him more than he needed to avoid it," Byock says. "That it really did matter more to us than him at that point. And so, he allowed it and it was really a gift to us." Byock has observed that when patients worry about creating more work or stress for their family, the family often tells him, "Oh no, no—we really want to take care of him."

I've caught glimpses of family members struggling as they've witnessed loved ones in this interval of living/dying, and their responses are usually imperfect. One man, apparently uncomfortable at the sight of his brother in a wheelchair, spent most of his visit on his cell phone. His brother only had a few days of life left, but he couldn't bring himself to put away the phone and just talk to him. In another case, a woman found one excuse after another to avoid visiting her dying sister until the last possible minute. Once there, she dissolved in tears, and then stayed only briefly.

I've also observed as a father started receiving calls from an estranged daughter every day after he was admitted to hospice. I was there when a man received two huge boxes of cookies from an elderly father with whom he'd lost contact. In general, people often seem to rise to the occasion. And as Byock observes, despite the burden and the difficulty, most of them *want* to care for their family members.

GROWING ACCUSTOMED TO THE LAND OF LIVING/DYING

I had to beg my mother to arrange her chemotherapy treatments around my teaching schedule so I could accompany her—not because she cared about which days she had the treatments, but because she didn't want to be a burden. Like so many other patients, my mother wanted to be treated as normally as possible, within the constrictions of her illness.

She wore a skirt and heels to the chemotherapy sessions, pre-serving her neat, poised exterior.

Who would have thought you could get used to sitting in a clinic for five hours with a bottle slowly dripping toxins into your veins? But people do, and my mother did, at least ap-parently. We would read together, or she would sleep and I'd grade papers; now and then, we'd talk about her cancer, about whether she was afraid of dying (*No*), what death might be like (*The thing that's hardest for me is imagining you all, my family, without me*), about how much we loved each other. Yet I think we also did a lot of pretending—my family for her, she perhaps for us—that she wasn't floating in an interval between life and death. And we were often too successful at the pretense.

Life in the land of living/dying isn't easy. It's also not nec-essarily unhappy or unrewarding. What the research shows is that life in this phase sometimes is exactly what any of us might expect—when and if we thought about it—but that in other aspects, it doesn't match our expectations and assump-tions at all.

That's also true of one of the circumstances that can make the biggest difference in our experience of the living/dying in-terval as well as the final, acute phase of dying: the place where we spend our last weeks and days.

chapter four
going home: where people die

IN EARLY 2005, my mother's chemo treatment—the latest in a series over the course of six years—ceased working. We met with her oncologist, who suggested she consider discontinuing chemotherapy. My mother went home and studied the remaining potential therapies and their long lists of potential side effects. She thought about her increasing weakness and the debilitating effects of some of the treatments—treatments that had grown less effective over time. She decided she'd had enough.

When we met with the oncologist again, my mother asked when we should start thinking about calling in hospice, and the doctor's answer caught us off guard: *Now.*

The news wasn't exactly shocking. Years before, a different oncologist had made it clear that my mother's cancer was incurable, although treatments could extend her life. Still, the moment in the doctor's office felt abrupt. Throughout her illness, it was as if we only knew how to converse about death in code. And now this new message was loud and clear: *"You're already eligible for hospice"* meant *"You are dying."*

As far as I know, my family hadn't discussed any of the nuts-and-bolts practicalities of death. My mother had said she only wanted to continue with treatments as long as her quality of life was good. We hadn't known what that point would be, or what the immediate implications might be. We hadn't talked about where her dying would happen, although I think we all assumed it would be at home.

WHERE DO YOU WANT TO DIE?

Joan Halifax asked a group of health professionals to describe their ideal death settings—to jot down where they would like to die.

Halifax, a Buddhist abbot who leads an annual seminar on "Being with Dying," is passionate about improving the experiences of dying people. She also intersperses her talks with stories from other parts of her life—six years of working with prisoners on death row, a marriage to psychiatrist Stanislav Grof in which they did joint research on psychedelic therapy for dying people, the time she realized she'd just delivered a lecture on compassion to the Dalai Lama.

Now, she asked the group for a show of hands: How many had said they wanted to die at home?

Almost everyone raised their hands.

What about at a favorite place, such as a family cabin or beachside cottage?

A few raised their hands.

Outdoors?

Two.

In a hospital or other institution?

No one raised a hand.

"But the fact is, many of us will die in a hospital or other institution," she said. While about 80 percent of Americans say they want to die at home, only 30 percent actually do, according to the CDC's most recent figures.

"You could say that's a failure," says Gary Rodin, the psychiatrist who works with advanced cancer patients. "And it is, in some cases, a failure to make plans so people can die at home. Certainly, if resources and planning are available, it's easier to die at home. But I think it's more a shift in perspective."

When people answer surveys about where they'd prefer to die, they're typically healthy. The question still feels hypothetical: "It's like asking, 'Would you want pain relief if you have a baby?'" Rodin explains. "If you ask somebody at the beginning of their pregnancy, they might have a different answer than at the time of delivery, because you're really just imagining what it would be like."

Even patients who only have a year left to live don't usually understand what's involved in dying, Rodin says. When people think about how and where they want to die, they tend to think they will have abilities and desires similar to those they have now. But the *you* who now believes dying at home is the best option may be very different from the *you* who is actively dying at some unknown point in the future. It's hard to know what your needs and wishes will be.

It's also hard to know in advance where you will actually spend your last days, whatever your wishes. A large national analysis of data about dying people in the 1990s, the SUP-PORT study, found that people's individual preferences about where they died made very little difference in where they actually died. Instead, it was the habit of the rest of their community that carried the most weight: If a local hospital had more available beds and most people in the community tended to die in the hospital, then no matter an individual patient's stated preferences, he was more likely to die in a hospital.

Barring a violent death or unforeseen accident, there are basically four settings where people die: in the hospital, at home, in a residential hospice, or in a nursing home.

THE ICU: WHY PEOPLE DON'T WANT
TO DIE IN HOSPITALS

Dying in the ICU is more likely to be painful than dying somewhere else, all things being equal, says Margaret Campbell, a professor of nursing at Wayne State University who has been working in palliative care for more than forty years: "[D]ying in an intensive care unit with full, aggressive use of life-sustaining therapy—that's all painful. Putting people on ventilators, putting tubes in, putting lines in—regardless of whether the underlying condition produces pain, the medicalization of trying to prevent dying is painful."

In the modern U.S. medical system for instance, *more* is almost always considered the right thing to do, says Jeremy Brown, the NIH emergency care director. If there's a chance of some small, incremental benefit in extending a patient's life, doctors are reluctant to *not* initiate treatments, even if you have a terminal disease and obviously have only a few days or weeks left.

I think one of the big differences within the United States in the nineteenth century was that 90 percent of lingering deaths—maybe even 95—would have been at home with family care. So I suspect that the people who were dying of decay, of old age, of mortification, of debility, would never have sought medical attention, or might have gotten the doctor's consult once. And the doctor would have said, "Yep, this person's old and dying—make him comfortable," and that would have been the end of it. Whereas, over the course of the twentieth century, all these deaths move into hospitals. Now people are trying to move them back out of hospitals. And surely, in the hospitals is where you start to get these concerns over extreme interventions

at death, and doctors who are refusing to let people go.
I don't think that had even been a consideration in the
nineteenth century.—DAVID JONES, HARVARD UNIVERSITY
PROFESSOR OF THE CULTURE OF MEDICINE

The most likely reason you'd land in a hospital emergency
room when you've known for a while that you're already close
to death is shortness of breath. And if a patient doesn't have
a clear advance directive—or if it's not readily available—
physicians will usually begin the same procedure they'd do
for anyone else. They'll insert a breathing tube and attach the
patient to a mechanical ventilator, or breathing machine.
For this procedure, physicians first sedate and paralyze the
patient. "You have to stop them from breathing because you
need the machine to take over, and if the patient is fighting the
machine and breathing on their own, it's difficult to get it in
sync," Brown explains. "Then you sort of tilt the head back and,
using a laryngoscope, which is a metal surgical device with a
long blade on it, you insert this breathing tube down the throat
of the patient through the larynx, the vocal cords, and then
it comes to rest just above where the two branches of the two
main bronchi divide. And then once you've got that in place, you
get a chest X-ray to make sure the tube is in the right place. You
listen to lung sounds to make sure that both sides are getting
oxygenated evenly, and you would then attach that patient, still
sedated, still paralyzed, to a breathing machine."

Inserting the breathing tube takes about five or ten minutes. It's usually effective both in increasing the amount of
oxygen in a patient's blood and addressing the patient's feeling of shortness of breath. But it's also invasive and can be
uncomfortable, and for someone who already has a fatal condition, the procedure introduces new problems and issues.

"By saying 'yes' to intubation, you're saying 'no' to a lot of
other things," Brown explains. "The first thing that you're

saying 'no' to by saying 'yes' to intubation, is saying 'no' to a patient being conscious and awake, and for a lot of people who are dying, that's an important thing. Their loved ones should be there, they have things that they might want to say, or they just do not want to be unconscious when that happens. So that's the first thing you're saying 'no' to.

"And the second thing you're saying 'no' to is the concept of death: You're essentially prolonging the inevitable." Intubations and other procedures medicalize death, Brown says: As soon as physicians insert a breathing tube, "the natural process of dying has been interfered with." If doctors hadn't stepped in and placed a patient on a breathing machine, the patient's oxygen would drop lower and lower until she drifted into unconsciousness. Her breathing would slow down, and then she would die.

But the breathing tube slows down that inevitable process. Once a dying person has a breathing tube, ICU staff and family members will probably have to decide whether or when to remove it. That's a hard decision because it involves taking an action to allow a dying person to finish the process of dying, rather than passively allowing it to happen.

Furthermore, patients on a ventilator can't be cared for anywhere else. Brown continues: "You are condemning them to the intensive care unit, where they are very likely to die, and a lot of people do not want to spend their last days in an intensive care unit. To many people, I suspect, dying at home is an extremely important, an extremely desired end—you're taking away that ability."

Of course, invasive procedures in the ICU are not the only kinds of hospital deaths. And someone with a terminal illness might prefer to die in a hospital for several reasons.

Sometimes, a Hospital Is the Best Place to Die
Hospitals offer a level of technology, equipment, expertise, and twenty-four-hour care not available at home or most in-

stitutions. And sometimes dying in a hospital is better than dying at home. Some symptoms can be burdensome, or even terrifying, for both patients and caregivers, or they're just too difficult to control at home. While hospice workers tend to have more specialized knowledge about dying than regular doctors or nurses, the medical staff at a hospital usually has a larger variety of specialized skills and expertise. Many hospices aren't set up to provide IVs to patients in their homes, so in cases of extreme pain, palliative care experts in hospitals can do a better job of treating the patient. More and more hospitals have units or doctors who specialize in palliative care, the discipline that focuses on pain and symptom management—and help with psychosocial, spiritual, and physical issues—for people who have an advanced illness. Hospice is a subset of palliative care, explains Anne Rossignol, who is both the palliative care doctor at Mercy Regional Medical Center, Durango's main hospital, and the doctor for Mercy Hospice House. All hospice is a kind of palliative care, but not all palliative care is hospice. Palliative care doctors are trained both in talking patients with advanced diseases through what their options are, and in treating symptoms like pain.

In an essay for *The Guardian*, Australian oncologist Ranjana Srivastava cites three cases in which patients said they wanted to die at home but ended up dying in a hospital. All three had terminated their curative treatments and were on palliative care. But when they reached their last days, they, or their family members, chose a hospital death. Srivastava offers this explanation:

> [T]here is one unmistakable thing that hospitals
> provide and patients clamour for—clinical expertise.
> There are caring nurses, vigilant doctors, continuous
> supervision and prompt symptom relief. There are

social workers and chaplains who can display calm
confidence in the face of challenges.

Hospitals are imperfect, she acknowledges. But they lift
the burden of care from family members and provide a higher
level of expertise. Maybe you still want to stay at home to die,
but that becomes unrealistic, Srivastava writes. Maybe you
don't have a caregiver at all. Maybe you simply change your
mind.

Even when caregivers are ready and willing, patients are
often deeply worried about becoming a burden. Or they value
the impersonal attentions of professionals. When three British
researchers examined cancer patients' preferences for place of
death, they found that "end of life care by professionals in an
institutional setting was certainly a preference for those patients who thought it 'not right' that a son, daughter or sibling
should be required to engage in intimate care tasks such as
toileting, bodily washing, or clearing up [feces] and vomit."

Until recently, most people in developed countries were dying in hospitals, but the trend is shifting. In the 1980s, the
number of Americans who died in acute care hospitals peaked
at about 54 percent—it reached 70 percent for patients dying
of cancer. The number has since dropped to 22 percent, as
hospice has allowed more people to remain at home or in a
nursing home to die.

HOME WITH HOSPICE

As a hospice volunteer, I've visited patients in their homes
more than in any other setting. When I knock on the door
the first time, I know a patient's name and condition, and little else. Each patient—and each patient's circumstances—is
unique. Here are a few:

- A fifty-year-old man who had no wife or children, and whose siblings lived far away. A neighbor agreed to be his primary caregiver so he could die at home.
- A woman who lived in her own home and was cared for by her relatives. Bits of trash littered the floors of the house, which was crammed with furniture and boxes of Christmas decorations in June. A chicken bone on the dresser next to her bed was still there when I returned a week later (I tossed it in the trash). The woman was eventually moved by Adult Protective Services to a nursing home.
- A man who lived with his wife in their comfortable and elegant home, its windows overlooking the town spread out below.
- A woman who lived in her own small apartment in an affordable housing complex. Her daughter was living with her temporarily but had to work during the day, so she patched together shifts of volunteer and privately paid caregivers to cover her times away.
- A woman who lived in a small home by herself, a stone's throw from her son and daughter-in-law's house on the same property.

Living out their last days at home wasn't easy for any of these people, but they and their families preferred it to the alternatives. In developed countries across the world, dying at home is just beginning to resurge after decades of hospitalizing dying people. Palliative care is a relatively new specialty, and in European countries with universal health care systems, the costs of palliative and hospice care may be easier for patients to bear. In the United States, Medicare is the primary payer, and its coverage of hospice made the choice to stay at home possible for my hospice patients and hundreds of thousands of others. Medicare is the primary payer for 85 percent of hospice patients, according to the latest figures available from the National Hospice and Palliative Care Organization. And ever since Congress ruled in 1983 that Medicare benefits should include hospice, the organization's role in the United States has largely been guided by Medicare and Medicaid.

To enroll, Medicare requires two doctors to certify that you have a life expectancy of six months or less, and that first step is a crux move that can prove daunting. It's hard to accept a fatal diagnosis, much less a date, no matter that the date is just an estimate. This step isn't easy for doctors, either. Prognoses tend to be inaccurate—they're usually too rosy—and it's often difficult to switch from talking optimistically with patients about cures and treatments, to counseling them about their impending deaths.

And Medicare has another vexing rule: Patients must agree not to seek further treatments aimed at extending their lives. My mother had already decided to stop her treatments before she asked about hospice, but for other patients, this requirement is often an additional hurdle. Even after a physician tells them they probably have six months or less to live, many patients aren't ready to stop seeking aggressive treatments. They're not ready to give up looking for a miracle cure. And that's a big part of why many people are reluctant to begin hospice until very close to death: because they see it as giving up.

Over time, this rule that hospice patients can't continue curative treatments—which is also followed by Medicaid and most private insurance plans—has softened. For instance, it is now possible to receive treatment that might have curative potential—radiation, say—if the main purpose of that treatment is to ease pain or other symptoms.

Also, signing up for hospice isn't final. Patients are reevaluated every sixty to ninety days and, now and then, some patients "graduate" from hospice, if a doctor believes their prognosis has improved significantly. You can stop hospice at any point, for any reason. If you change your mind and decide you still want to try another clinical trial or curative treatment, you can leave hospice. And you can also return. Forty percent of hospice patients use the service for two weeks or less, according to the most recent figures from the National Hospice and Palliative Care Organization. Using hospice for only a few days means patients don't receive most of the benefits—the more specialized attention to pain treatment and symptoms, the social and emotional support, or the continuous care under one main medical entity, for instance.

"To really get it right, you need more than three days of hospice," says Joan Teno, the University of Washington professor whose research focuses on end-of-life care and policy issues. When dying patients *are* admitted to hospice, families report that dying at home under hospice care is the best-case scenario, Teno says. A national study she coauthored found that family members were twice as likely to rate care for dying patients as excellent if hospice had been involved.

In hindsight, I don't remember ever consciously choosing where my mother would die: She would remain at home, of course. She had plenty of family and more than enough friends to take care of her at home, and she had breast cancer—a disease whose steady progress makes it easier to know when to stop pursuing last-ditch efforts in the hospital. Like the majority of hospice patients and families I've talked with, hospice care at home was a good choice for her. Families often give glowing reports about hospice staff members: *They've been so wonderful,* they'll say, faces radiating gratitude. *Everyone— the nurses, the social workers, the volunteers.* But, of course, hospice is not perfect. Furthermore, what it offers or does not offer, and what it requires, can catch people by surprise.

HOW HOSPICE WORKS

Hospice usually begins within a couple of days of a doctor's referral. "I'm the one that's usually telling somebody, 'You talked to your doctor today, and I'm sorry you have this prognosis,'" says Michelle Appenzeller, the clinical director at Hospice of Mercy in Durango. She always tells the person, "I'm sorry I had to meet you this way. It's a tough time. I'm going to help you get through, and this is what to expect."

A nurse or social worker shows up at your home and, together, you figure out what you want or need, and what hospice can provide. You receive pain medications—and pain management is an area in which most hospices excel.

If you need it, hospice will provide equipment like a wheelchair, an oxygen tank, or a bedside commode. You get a hospital bed, if you want one. When the hospice nurse first mentioned the hospital bed to my family, we looked askance and we initially refused—after all, why wouldn't she want to sleep in the comfortable bed she had selected herself long ago, the one she shared with my father? The nurse just nodded and said it would be available if my mother wanted it later. Eventually, the hospital bed made it easier for her to sit up and lie down. And while losing each other was heartbreaking, my parents by then were drifting into different spheres: my father still busily engaging in society; she, slipping into the world of the dying. In this case, hospice staff knew better than we did what we would need, but they also knew to wait until we were ready.

You, the patient, get to decide which hospice services you need. You have access to a team of caregivers: nurses, home health aides, social workers, a physician, a chaplain, and volunteers to assist with tasks like light housekeeping or dishes—or just being there when caregivers need a break. The interdisciplinary team is one of the most important elements of hospice, says Fred Schwartz, the medical director of Hospice New York. Through its interdisciplinary team, hospice focuses on more than the physical dimension, Schwartz says. "We're taking care of a person's emotional needs, their social needs . . . Or, what are the dynamics of that patient's life, in a social way? And certainly in a spiritual, metaphysical way? What is going on when somebody has to leave this plane of reality, and who am I going to talk to about that?" Hospice is not just for the person with a terminal diagnosis. "It's for the whole family, whatever that family concept is—significant other, a friend, traditional family, children, grandchildren," Schwartz says. "Whatever that dynamic is, where the patient is, together with other people in the community, we work with them."

But the essence of hospice care, for many people, is the availability of nurses and nurses' aides. They're accustomed to dealing with death; they're usually knowledgeable about how to make dying people more comfortable and at ease. Nurses are on call twenty-four hours a day and will visit in the middle of the night if necessary. They see hospice patients at their homes one to three times a week. Home health aides provide additional visits—in New York that can be as frequently as five days a week, although New York is unusually generous in this area.

"But what really, truly surprises people is that we're not going to be there 24/7," Appenzeller says. Neither hospice nurses nor aides are present twenty-four hours a day, and this is the beginning of another difficult truth about hospice: For the most part, hospice does not provide around-the-clock care. There are rare exceptions—patients in a crisis may have continuous home care for very brief periods, for instance. Medicare will also pay for respite care. Respite in this case is for caregivers, in the form of a few days every billing cycle when patients are temporarily transferred to a nursing home or hospital.

Because hospice doesn't typically provide day care, most hospice patients who stay at home need to have their own caregiver of some kind. In many cases, this is a joyful duty for family members. However, it can be difficult or impossible for a spouse with physical limitations or in cases where family members have to be gone for work regularly. And because some patients live alone, the lack of round-the-clock care can prove an obstacle to dying at home with hospice.

This particular hospice framework, which generally assumes patients will have their own caregivers, could have been different. After all, it was originally modeled on the famous St. Christopher's hospice in London founded by the British doctor Cicely Saunders as a place where patients would stay and be tended by nurses for twenty-four hours a day.

A QUICK HISTORY OF HOSPICE

Saunders was first inspired by her work with dying people at other hospices in London. So it made sense that her efforts focused on creating a place, St. Christopher's, where she could implement her research and methods to help patients. Residential hospices—places where dying patients go and stay and are provided with palliative care—still offer a significant percentage of care for dying people in Great Britain.

That was also the case in the United States in the early 1970s, when hospices were first being established here, says James Hallenbeck, who has written a history of the Veterans Affairs hospices: "At that time, almost all [hospices] were inpatient units, very much like St. Christopher's in England."

But hospice in the United States and in Great Britain would travel distinctly different routes: British hospices are run and maintained by the government, through the National Health Service. In the United States, Medicare or Medicaid pays the majority of hospice costs, but they never run the organizations. American hospices may be overseen by private hospitals or nonprofits or, increasingly, they may be for-profit organizations.

In the ferment of conflicting visions and practicalities as American hospices were forming, anti-institutional ideas and concerns about costs coalesced. People envisioned hospice as a way for more people to die at home, and so the Medicare benefit did not include room and board (although Hallenbeck points out that Veterans Affairs hospices remain the exception—these have all remained residential). Hospice in the United States, for the most part, evolved into a specific kind of care, rather than a place.

There are still some residential hospices in the United States, and more hospitals are adding special hospice wings or sections. In Durango, Colorado, for instance, Mercy Hospice has just built a $5.6 million, state-of-the-art hospice facility with eight beds. The building is idyllic: There are spacious private bedrooms, a meditation room, a kitchen for family and friends, and sitting rooms where people can visit in private.

I believe the significant difference between Hospice House and the home program is that in the Hospice House, you are really involved in all aspects of the family and the patients—the good, the bad and the ugly. In the home program, for example, when somebody calls and there's some kind of an issue or problem, you call the social worker, they go into the home, they're there for an hour, and then they're gone. In the Hospice House, it never stops.

So, for example, on Friday, there was a family and it was very complicated. There are so many players, and you have to figure out who all the players are, and then who should get access. I hear the story, and the chaplain hears the story, and the social worker hears the story, and then I call the social worker. And she comes in and

*then Family One is saying one thing, but we have to keep
Family Two away, because Family One is the guardian.
And the chaplain is saying, "Family Two is also a bona
fide family," and I'm saying, "Yeah, it's bona fide all
right—but it has no legal right, because the guardian
says no."*

*In the home, you walk away. Even though you might
be in there two hours; you walk away; it's done. You
don't know, if after three o'clock "Bad Family" is going
in. At Hospice House, you know everything, because the
families are always there. You get to know them; it's
a whole different relationship. It is a whole different
relationship.* —MICHELLE APPENZELLER, CLINICAL DIRECTOR
AT DURANGO'S HOSPICE OF MERCY

Until recently, the Zen Hospice Guest House in San Francisco offered another kind of residential hospice. Founded by
Buddhists shortly after the AIDS crisis began in 1987, it eventually was turned into a separate nonprofit organization. The
two-story Victorian house could seem unorthodox for a medical setting—a temperamental elevator was the only alterna-
tive to steep stairs, for instance—but a nurse and nurse's
aide were on site 24/7, and the environment was comfortable
and homelike. With a kitchen staff that prepared individual
meals-to-order and where the smell of baking pastries often
permeated the living room, the Zen hospice seemed nearly
perfect. But its six beds were seldom full and in the spring
of 2018, the hospice stopped accepting patients. The building
was sold that autumn.

For both the San Francisco and the Durango residential
hospices, the catch is that charges for room and board are not
covered by Medicare, Medicaid, or most private insurances.
The organizations work with patients and often charge on a

sliding scale, but for many people, residential hospices are simply not an affordable or available option.

That's one of the reasons that 70 percent of hospices in the United States are now home based. Which still sounds preferable to dying in an institution, and is, in many ways. When dying patients received home hospice care, their families' needs were met better than other families', according to a study Teno coauthored. And it's just common sense that patients are usually more comfortable in the familiar environment of their homes, says Peter Rogatz, the former director of the Long Island Jewish Medical Center and a cofounder of End of Life Choices New York. Furthermore, caregivers are more likely to be able to respond quickly and intuitively to their needs: "When you're at home, whether you're in hospice or just in general home care, the person who's responsible for giving you your meds—your spouse, your cousin, your daughter—is much more interested in being sure that you get your medications on time, that you're not in pain, that if you need a bed pan, that you're getting it when you need it and not half-an-hour later."

There are exceptions. A British researcher, Kristian Pollock, points out that for some patients, dying at home may lead to inadequate care: "Just because a death occurred at home does not mean that it was good. The person may have been alone, inadequately supported, in pain, distressed, and fearful. Idealised [sic] accounts of 'the good death' at home often do not recognise the reality of intractable pain and discomfort experienced by some dying patients and, for a substantial number, the sheer hard work of dying." If you have a chronic, debilitating illness and long periods when you're dependent on others, you're more likely to die in some kind of institution, writes Hallenbeck. And, under those circumstances, that may be a better death.

TRANSITIONS

For patients hoping to avoid aggressive treatment at the end of life, a 2010 report from the CDC seemed to offer good news: It stated that significantly more people were dying at home rather than in hospitals, and hospice and palliative care use was growing. A study of cancer patient deaths showed the United States had the lowest number of deaths in the hospital out of seven developed countries. The researchers concluded that "end-of-life care can evolve to reflect patient preferences and goals about site of death."

But Teno points out that where people are at the moment they die doesn't tell the whole story. She and her colleagues examined Medicare records that showed where people stayed, not just the last day but the last three months, before they died. They found that 11 percent of the patients they studied had three or more hospitalizations in the last ninety days of life. Furthermore, the number of moves in the last seventy-two hours of patients' lives rose by 36 percent between 2000 and 2009, the time period Teno and her colleagues studied.

Teno calls it "the old hot potato game": The earlier an institution is able to send a patient home or to the next institution, the more money the institution saves because Medicare reimburses medical providers a set amount per patient, rather than according to the amount of time patients spend in an institution. "Everybody's handing off these people, and no one's really focusing on the entire experience and making sure it goes smoothly," she says.

Most importantly, the number of transitions is hard on patients, Teno says: "When you make all those transitions, it's very difficult for the patient, for the family."

In a different study, Teno and her coauthors note that while more Americans are dying at home and fewer people are dying in hospitals, the number of people dying in nursing homes was creeping up.

NURSING HOMES*

"[C]ontradictory to the common stereotype, dying in a nursing home is not the worst scenario," writes researcher Siew Tzuh Tang, who conducted a study on where terminally ill cancer patients prefer to die. "On the contrary, a nursing home may be most appropriate and desired for a segment of terminally ill patients."

As a hospice volunteer—patients in nursing homes can also enroll in hospice—I've sometimes found that to be true. Here are some of the hospice patients I've visited at nursing homes:

- A man who lived alone in a comfortable assisted living facility. He spent most of the day watching television in his small living room.
- A woman who lived in an assisted-living suite with her husband, who was still healthy. They sat in easy chairs together in their shared living room during much of the day. When she had trouble sleeping at night, he moved into the second bedroom in their suite. After she stopped cooking or eating much, he could easily walk down the hallway to the cafeteria for his meals.
- A man who lived in a nursing home, with no friends or family visiting. He had a rare form of Parkinson's disease that reduced his vocabulary to the single word, "No." Staff members didn't like him. One aide told me the man would eat his napkin at meals if not closely monitored, and that he'd once tried to swallow the telephone handset at the nurses' station.

---

* While nursing homes and assisted living facilities are very different from each other and are governed by different sets of regulations, the terms are used almost interchangeably here to refer to the homes and institutions for people who have some type of disability or need long-term care or assistance.

While nursing home stays sometimes drain a family's savings, they can also be an affordable option, depending on several factors. In the United States, if patients have been hospitalized for at least three days and need skilled nursing, Medicare will pay 100 percent of the costs of a nursing home for up to twenty days. After that, Medicare will help to pay the costs for an additional eighty days if necessary, but patients are expected to co-pay.

Medicaid, although it varies from state to state, pays for approximately 64 percent of all nursing home patients. But its rules usually require people to first exhaust most of their savings, and then pay almost all their remaining income to Medicaid. The silver lining is that once patients fulfill these requirements, they no longer have to pay for meals, lodging, or nursing care.

Those basic benefits made a big impact for my hospice patient who started out being cared for at home by her relatives: The patient, who was one hundred years old and had dementia, weighed about ninety pounds on good days, and hospice staff members were concerned about her diet and basic hygiene. After the patient was moved to a nursing home, she gained weight and she talked more—and she has survived far longer than nurses had expected.

For some patients, nursing homes offer the prospect of a safer environment than their own homes, with a chance at greater control and personalization than hospitals. Most skilled nursing facilities also provide a strong social component: daily scheduled activities, meals in a communal setting, and visits from schoolchildren, choirs, and pet therapy volunteers. An eighty-year-old with lung cancer told Tang there were opportunities for friendships because patients tended to stay longer there than they did in hospitals. And he described other advantages: "The nursing home has a more homelike environment than a hospital. Staying in a nursing home, I may have my own 'territory.' I can decorate my room with the pictures of my family." Despite the benefits, most dying people say they hope to avoid nursing homes at all costs. Questions about nursing homes in interviews evoked an "only as a last resort" response, even in cases where standards of care were known to be good. When an interviewer asked one patient about her feelings regarding dying in a nursing home, the patient responded with laughter: "Oh, shut up—for goodness' sake . . . Oh God, I hope I don't need that, ever."

This patient, like another in the same study, was most concerned about being surrounded chiefly by elderly people, especially patients with dementia.

Nursing homes may have other issues, such as understaffing and high turnover rates. Nursing home patients who are on hospice are less likely to receive hospice nurse visits than patients receiving care elsewhere. Their families report they are less likely to be treated with respect, and more likely to have untreated pain.

Medicare and Medicaid have introduced policy changes that can provide more funding for hospice visits in the last week of a person's life, Teno says. She's also hopeful that many of the problems affecting dying people in nursing homes can be addressed through thoughtful staff education.

What makes Teno most hopeful, however, is a trend away from an emphasis on where dying patients stay. Organizations now tend to be reimbursed on a volume-based incentive system. But Teno believes the United States is moving toward a value-based system, one "that looks at the patient experience, not just the experience in the hospital, the experience in the nursing home, and the experience of home health." Instead, the new system will focus on how a patient intersects with all three of these settings, which will have "shared account-ability" for what happens to patients. "So, I'm optimistic," she says. "I hope we can get it right."

WHERE WE DIE MATTERS, BUT MAYBE WE HAVE LESS CONTROL OVER IT THAN WE THINK

When people are asked their preferences about where they'd most like to die, some researchers warn that the answers are not as clear-cut as they seem. There's rarely an option for "it depends," or "it doesn't matter," writes Pollock, the British researcher, in her analysis about whether home really is the preferred place of death. The idea that we have a choice about where—or how—we die, can be misleading. Factors such as the kind of illness, severity of symptoms, availability of resources, and amount of caregiver support may make that choice for us. "We might ask if the notion of 'choice' applies to death: most people would prefer, presumably, to be not ill, not old, not dying," she writes.

Other people seem to believe that patients have a right to decide where and how they die, she writes, but "patients often have a more cautious and circumspect approach, suggesting a pragmatic and more realistic appraisal of uncertainty, as well as apprehension, about how they will respond to the unfathomable experience of dying."

You also may not be fully aware as you approach death. I think of one hospice patient, a fifty-three-year-old man who had glioblastoma, an aggressive cancer in the brain. Although his wife was taking care of him at home and could afford paid caregivers, she was sometimes overwhelmed. So the patient came for multiple respite stays at a hospice residence. He was a sweet man, but his mind had been affected by the cancer: He was convinced he was working in some sort of engineering job at hospice, and he would stare at his cell phone for fifteen or twenty minutes as if he were reading important messages, although the phone was turned off. After ordering his dinner one night, he carefully placed it in a communal freezer down the hall, and then dumped all of his magazines, coloring books, and markers into a trash can when I wasn't looking. He was driven by a restless energy to pace for hours, and despite his poor balance and the cold outside temperatures, he would often try to escape through the exterior doors, so either a volunteer or nurse's aide would walk the halls with him, endlessly pacing the corridors.

Once, I visited him at his home, where he also roamed from room to room, climbing up and down the stairs, trying the handles of all the doors to the outside. Eventually, he was admitted to full-time care at the hospice house, where he gradually stopped roaming and slept more and more until he died. At both his home and the hospice house, this man lived in very comfortable style, with attentive care, good food, nice furnishings. At both places, he seemed miserable much of the time, and I wonder whether the *where* mattered to him.

Where you die can very much matter in determining *how* you die, however. Rossignol says she predicted the following scenario for her elderly mother, who had very advanced dementia: "She's going to fall and break her hip, and then we're going to get her on hospice, and then she's going to die." Sure enough, some months later, Rossignol's mother fell and broke her hip. Rossignol lived in another state, but she called the emergency department where she had once worked: "We're not going to call the orthopedic doctors," Rossignol told the ER doctor, a friend of hers. There would be no curative treatments, no attempts to fix the hip. "We're going to get her comfortable. Give her lots of pain medicines. I'm on my way." Rossignol then called her hospice friends. "Here we come," she told them. Nine days later, Rossignol's mother died, surrounded by family. "But I've got to tell you, there were lots of days that I wondered, 'Am I doing the right thing?'" Rossignol confessed. "She's my *mom,* right?"

Rossignol's best guess is that her mother would have *thought* she would prefer to have treatment and go to a nursing home, but the actual experience would have been terrible. She would have been content for the one or two hours a day when she received attentive care. "And then the rest of the twenty-two hours a day, she would have been lonely and miserable," Rossignol says.

"I know we did the right thing," Rossignol says. "It's not easy; it's never easy—I told one of my patients' family members that today: 'It's never easy.'"

chapter five
does dying hurt?

THREE DAYS BEFORE my mother died, her pain medications suddenly stopped working. She was unconscious or semiconscious, but the pain half lifted her from her pillows and she shuddered with convulsions. For hours, nothing—not extra doses of morphine or calls to the doctor or a different drug added to the mix she was already taking—seemed to diminish the pain.

By the evening, my mother finally seemed calm and comfortable, but my family was shaken by the episode.

This experience is not uncommon. A 2015 study compares two surveys of dying patients' families, conducted ten years apart. The study finds that the experience of dying in the United States has grown worse, at least according to the families' perceptions. A key part of the study is family observations of patients' pain. In the first survey, 15.5 percent of the family members said the dying patient had needed more pain management than he or she received. In the second survey, that number had risen to 25 percent.

In an even larger study of family member reports, researchers interviewed family members from 1998 to 2010 about their relatives' dying experiences. Half reported that dying patients had experienced moderate or significant pain. When other researchers interviewed patients with terminal diseases directly, they also found that 50 percent reported moderate or serious pain.

Unless something changes, then, about half of us can expect to experience serious pain at some point during our final months or weeks. But is this a systemic failure, something that medical progress or social reforms might change? Or is pain somehow an intrinsic part of dying?

DYING DOES INVOLVE SUFFERING, BUT . . .

Many palliative care specialists insist that some physical or psychological or spiritual distress is unavoidable: Parts of dying *will* cause suffering. "We're losing everything that we've loved," explains Ira Byock, the former hospice doctor who writes about dying. "We're losing life itself; we're losing all of our relationships, all of our possessions."

Furthermore, pain is not the only kind of physical suffering dying people experience. As your body shuts down, you might have trouble breathing. You might have a severe cough or painful bedsores, or endure constipation or nausea. Still, James Hallenbeck, the palliative care expert, says, "We've gotten quite good about treating pain, shortness of breath, constipation, itching, all sorts of stuff—not perfect, but for most people physically, it's pretty easy."

Whether or not it *is* controlled, most physical pain associated with dying *can* be controlled, Hallenbeck says. "The number of really, really, bad, 'can't-fix-it' pain syndromes I've seen is a tiny handful. For physical pain, we're pretty good."

Fred Schwartz, the medical director of Hospice New York, says that's been true in his experiences with hospice patients: "Maybe 98 percent of the time, we can control the patient's pain at home." One of the main reasons is the availability of more powerful medications that are easy to administer, such as fentanyl patches. In addition, for patients who can no longer swallow, morphine and other medications in liquid form or a rapidly dissolving tablet can be placed under the patient's tongue: "So it's not that hard for family members now to administer pain medication in ways that we didn't have twenty, thirty years ago," Schwartz says.

Hallenbeck says the problem is often that pain is undertreated: The means exist to control a patient's pain, but somehow, somewhere along the way, that doesn't always happen.

PAIN ISN'T ALL IN YOUR HEAD—BUT MUCH OF IT IS

Pain is complicated.

People tend to imagine it as traveling a direct path from the senses to the brain. You twist your ankle and your brain immediately tells you: *Ouch.* But that's not how it works. The way you experience pain is closer to the way physician Atul Gawande describes human perception in a 2008 essay in *The New Yorker*:

> The images in our mind are extraordinarily rich. We can tell if something is liquid or solid, heavy or light, dead or alive. But the information we work from is poor—a distorted, two-dimensional transmission with entire spots missing. So the mind fills in most of the picture.

That is, perception isn't a window directly onto the world. Instead, it's more like "the brain's best guess about what is happening in the outside world," Gawande writes.

Likewise, your experience of pain might be described as your brain's best guess about whether something's hurting your body, and how concerned you should be. Pain is always filtered through the brain's complex understanding of what the signal your nerves send represents, including the past (How does it compare to earlier experiences?) and the future

(How long will it last?) and the actual threat (Could it represent a fatal injury?).

As a thought experiment, Hallenbeck says he's pictured someone asking him to rate his pain when he's under the drill in a dentist's chair. He figures his answer would usually be a two or three; his pain is well controlled by lidocaine and he knows the drilling won't last. "But if someone came up to me and said, 'You know, whatever it is you're experiencing, you're going to experience that for the rest of your life,'" his answer would be entirely different. He'd rate the pain as unbearable.

Hallenbeck knows he would experience the physical pain differently based on his mental projections, which is a factor in how much something hurts anyone. The International Association for the Study of Pain says pain "is always a psychological state, even though we may well appreciate that pain most often has a proximate physical cause. Pain is always subjective."

That means the amount of pain a person feels, and how much that person suffers, is very individual. "Pain is not only a sensation," writes Eric Cassell, the author of a classic book about pain and suffering, *The Nature of Suffering and the Goals of Medicine*. "It is also an experience embedded in beliefs about causes and diseases and their consequences."

Sometimes, I would be really aggressive with increasing a patient's pain dose, and it wasn't helping. And then I would be like, "Duh, maybe there's something else going on here." And I'd get the chaplain in, or I'd get the social worker to talk with them. And it turned out there was a whole other thing.—MARIAN GRANT, HOSPICE AND PALLIATIVE CARE NURSE PRACTITIONER

It's not that pain is "just psychological," or that you might easily rethink your way to overcoming pain. The fact that pain is always subjective doesn't make it any less real, but it has affected how we think about it and how effectively physicians control it. Cassell describes the case of a sixteen-year-old patient who had his knee replaced: After surgery, the patient was told that if his pain didn't diminish, surgeons "would have to revise his knee." When his pain continued to increase and proved unresponsive to opioids, the patient was hospitalized. Only then did medical professionals learn that he had misunderstood their explanation: He had thought that *revising* meant *amputating* his knee. "When he discovered that amputation was not in anybody's thoughts except his, pain control became simple," Cassell writes. The patient's physical pain didn't disappear, but his suffering diminished significantly when his understanding of what the pain meant became less threatening.

Another patient Cassell describes believed the severe pain in her leg was being caused by sciatica. Small doses of codeine were enough to treat the pain, but then she learned her leg was actually hurting because her disease was spreading. Suddenly, she needed much larger doses of medication to find any relief.

"Pain is not suffering . . . and pain relief, although vitally important, is not the relief of suffering," Cassell writes. Suffering, he explains, is something else: It's distress that threatens someone's sense of personhood—including elements like a person's future or past, relationships with others, culture, spirituality, and needs to find work and meaning. Severe, acute pain almost always causes suffering, but more minor pains may cause equal amounts of suffering. People's actual experience of physical pain usually causes more suffering "when they feel out of control, when the pain is overwhelming, when the source of the pain is unknown, when the meaning of the pain is dire, or when the pain is apparently without end."

Cicely Saunders, the hospice pioneer, realized early that the complexity of pain had practical implications in treating dying people. When she first began working as a nurse in London in the 1940s, she was moved by the unnecessary misery and suffering so many dying patients endured. She noticed that doctors would wait until patients cried out in pain before they administered medication. Once patients received a fatal diagnosis, they were often basically abandoned by medical workers, who felt they could no longer do anything for them.

Saunders—who after working as a nurse became a social worker and, eventually, a physician—began advocating to keep pain under continual control. She studied treatments for physical pain, developing a sophisticated and nuanced understanding of drugs that were available at the time. She believed in the importance of individualized protocols, and she learned that it was just as crucial to consider mental and emotional pain, which she called "perhaps the most intractable pain of all." Saunders famously focused on treating "total pain," which included mental, physical, spiritual, and social aspects of a patient's experience, and modern hospices in the United States have built on this concept.

But that doesn't mean they're always able to keep pain under control. For one thing, only patients can say how much they're hurting.

CALCULATING PAIN

There's no instrument like a thermometer or stethoscope for measuring pain in the way that other vital signs are measured. Instead, the best way to measure pain has always been to ask patients about it, most commonly by having them rate their pain on a scale of 1 to 10. But the pain scale doesn't work in the same way as, say, an oxygen saturation meter, which is used to measure the amount of oxygen in your blood.

At best, the scale is an approximation. Most people are

in rough agreement: "From about a one to four, for example, they're saying, 'I'm in some pain,' but they can kind of handle it," Hallenbeck explains. "Somewhere between a three and a four and a five, they're saying, 'I could use something for it,' and at a five, six, or seven or eight—somewhere in that range—they're communicating, 'I want something right away.'"

But Hallenbeck has seen enough patients to know that some people seem to live on completely different scales. He tells the story of a patient who said his pain was a 1.2 on a scale of 1 to 10. Hallenbeck wasn't sure what to make of that degree of precision, given the scale's inexactness. He says the rest of his exchange with the patient went something like this:

"Okay—do you need anything for that?"

"No, I don't think I need anything more for that."

"How much would it take for you to need something?"

"About a 1.89."

Doctors often have to rely on good guesswork when they're trying to figure out how much pain medication to prescribe. Complicating matters is the fact that patients will sometimes co-opt pain measurements. Nessa Coyle, the nurse researcher, noticed the way patients would adjust their pain reports depending on the situation, often in very sophisticated ways. If you're a patient with a fatal disease, you might observe a doctor's response to your past pain ratings and adjust accordingly, she says. Your calculations might take into account the amount of pain you've experienced in the past, the amount of relief you've received for that pain, and the methods used to treat it—as well as the side effects of those treatments. Then, you'd basically do a cost-benefit analysis to decide how much pain to admit to. One patient who under-reported the pain he experienced told Coyle: "I accepted the pain because I wanted to receive the experimental chemotherapy. I figured that if they treated me for pain I wouldn't be eligible for the drug."

Some patients under-report pain for other reasons, Hallenbeck says. Cancer patients have told him they don't *want* their pain to completely disappear; they ask him not to try to get it down to zero on the pain scale: "If it went to zero, how would I know what that cancer's doing in there?" patients have told him. "The pain is a way of the cancer talking to me, and I know if I totally wiped it out, I wouldn't know what was going on in there. I want it to be at a one or a two, because that way I can keep an eye on it."

The ways in which pain is experienced and reported make it difficult to treat, but even when patients and doctors share a good understanding, the medications available for treatment are far from flawless. And, like pain itself, the drugs are embedded in cultural beliefs and contexts that add layers of complexity.

A RELUCTANCE TO USE STRONG PAIN MEDS

The gold standard for treating acute pain for hundreds of years has been, and remains, some form of opium. Opioids, which mimic natural substances in the body but are more powerful, bind to opioid receptors in the brain and elsewhere, blocking pain signals—sometimes completely. They calm a person's emotional response to pain and cause a release of dopamine. For dying patients who are suffering, the drugs can be very effective, but they are often underused.

Joan Teno, who coauthored the study on dying patients' families' reports, recalls a time when she was serving as proxy decision maker for a patient. The patient was in extreme pain but wasn't receiving enough medication, so Teno fired the doctor and transferred the patient to hospice. "It was a physician who basically just didn't know how to provide good end-of-life care," she says. "He was afraid to use opiates."

A doctor afraid to use opiates?

"For someone who doesn't prescribe a lot of opiates, there's always sort of that background concern . . . that their patient's going to get addicted," she says.

An average family doctor probably only sees about three or four deaths a year, out of perhaps a thousand patients, she estimates. "It's a very small number of patients for that individual doctor. And so, for the most part, he's not used to having to handle people who are actively dying." That kind of unfamiliarity with dying can lead to undertreatment of pain by medical professionals, especially because of fears about using powerful drugs.

One of the unspoken rules nurses have about pain medication is that they should try to avoid being the nurse who gives the last dose of pain medicine, Teno says. "People worry that, 'I'm going to kill the patient with morphine,' but there are very good studies that if you follow the guidelines, you're not going to kill someone with morphine."

Studies show that doctors sometimes delay giving dying patients morphine—and therefore relief from pain—because of the following logical fallacy: Because morphine is so often prescribed to dying people, the morphine must be partly *responsible* for those deaths. It's not, of course, but the association lingers. That can also be true for patients and family members. Because opioids are so commonly used to treat pain in dying patients, most people have known someone who was started on morphine and then died not long after, so morphine and death are often closely linked in their minds. The mere mention of morphine is sometimes deeply disturbing to patients themselves or to their family members.

People are also afraid of taking or prescribing morphine because they're worried about becoming addicted. The current opioid epidemic is the worst in U.S. history: 115 people a day die from an opioid overdose in the United States, and most of those deaths involve prescriptions at some point, according to a 2018 report by the National Institutes of Health. While American opioid numbers dwarf those in most other countries, the crisis is rising across the globe. And fears about opioid addiction existed long before the latest upsurge. The addictive powers of opium played a role in colonial exploitation and were a leading factor in the two Opium Wars between England and China in the 1800s. Opioid addiction was also a serious problem for soldiers returning from the Civil War in the United States and both world wars. Early on, researchers began trying to create a perfect opioid, some sort of nonaddictive morphine. One solution they came up with was heroin, introduced in 1898 by the Bayer Company in Germany, but "by 1910, young working-class Americans had learned to crush the pills into powder and inhale it to achieve a concentrated high," writes Marcia Meldrum in an article about the history of treating pain. "The frightening spread in street use, coupled with rising alarm over iatrogenic addiction to morphine [addiction caused by medical treatment], encouraged the medical profession's support of the Harrison Narcotic Control Act, passed in 1914."

But studies show that addiction is rarely an issue for people diagnosed with a fatal condition. Hallenbeck says one reason for patients' apprehensions about opioids is that they fail to realize the difference between the ways in which doctors and abusers administer the drugs. "The part that kills people with opioids is the rate of rise of the opioid," he says. An addict who takes too rapid a dose to get high might be killed when it shuts down his respiratory system. "That's not how we use opioids," he says. "Yes, they are dangerous drugs, particularly if they're used by people who aren't skilled in their use. Used skillfully, there are a whole lot more dangerous drugs out there."

PAIN MEDICATIONS HAVE SIDE EFFECTS

Even without the stigma of potential addiction, opioids and other medications would still be a flawed solution to pain.

Hallenbeck says he's had something like the following conversation more than once:

> A common complaint, both from patients and families, is, "I just want Dad to have a great night's sleep and wake up totally alert at seven thirty every morning the way he did."
> My response is, "I wish we knew how to do that. I'm pretty damn good at what I do—I'm not that good. I don't know anyone else who is."
> We can't just put people—poof!—deep asleep, and then—poof!—wide awake. Our drugs are imperfect. So part of the dialogue around sleep, and it's similar around pain, is, "Help me understand the balance here. I can give them something more to help them sleep, but the cost will probably, given our current technology, mean they're going to be fuzzyheaded in the morning, or maybe a little more confused. I don't know how you value those things. Tell me where your balance is, and then we'll work it out together."

Treating pain is always a balancing act, he says. "We can get everybody under control if we just anesthetize them. But there are side effects to that."

Patients need to think in terms of trade-offs, says Marian Grant, the hospice and palliative care nurse practitioner. Opioids almost always cause constipation, so often that medications to treat that constipation are usually prescribed in concert with the drugs. They may also cause nausea or slight confusion or sleepiness, depending on the dose. And they can interact with other medications the patient may be taking.

Studies show that patients are often reluctant to start opioids because they're concerned about those side effects. They're usually most worried about constipation, and about remaining alert. Like Hallenbeck, Grant says she tells her patients, "I can control your pain, but you might be more sleepy." She'll describe a continuum with extreme alertness and pain at one end, and unconsciousness and a complete lack of pain at the other, and ask patients, "Where on that continuum are you willing to be?" Some tell her they'd rather be sleepy than awake and in pain. Other people say it's important to remain awake and alert, even if that means dealing with significantly more pain. "It's just a negotiation about what's important to them and what can I do," she says.

TIMING MATTERS

When my mother was enrolled in hospice, she was prescribed oxycodone for the pain, along with medications for the side effects. But in the first few days, she was still sometimes overwhelmed by pain and exhaustion and would melt onto the couch or her bed. After a family friend gently scolded us for not helping her keep track of all the pills—we hadn't realized that my mother would miss doses entirely, or she'd fail to take enough pills, so she had fallen behind in controlling her pain—my family jumped in, but it took a few days to catch up with her pain.

In the 1980s, the World Health Organization became so concerned about undertreated pain that it developed a set of guidelines for treating cancer pain. The key component was a stepladder of recommended treatments. If patients weren't in extreme pain, medical professionals were to begin treatments with non-opioids such as aspirin and acetaminophen. If pain persisted, they moved up a step in intensity by administering weak opioids such as codeine. Finally, if pain still wasn't under control, patients were to receive strong opioids such as morphine.

One important element of those guidelines was a recommendation that drugs be administered "by the clock," meaning in regular doses, rather than as needed. When a person has to wait until pain returns for more medication, it can take time to get the pain back under control. Also, patients may be too weak or confused to say something about increased pain. In contrast, the "by-the-clock" method means a drug is given at regular intervals, theoretically staying ahead of the pain. Under normal circumstances, it takes somewhere around a half hour or forty minutes for most analgesics to take effect, but when dying patients are already in severe pain by the time they're admitted to the hospital or hospice, it might require more time—hours or a couple of days—to relieve that pain adequately. If a patient is in a crisis—her pain is at 10 out of 10—it also may take more skill to treat that pain rapidly and safely, as doctors negotiate the balance between addressing pain quickly and avoiding extreme side effects. Even once pain is generally under control, patients still may experience "breakthrough pain"—sudden, intense spikes. These can be triggered by moving a patient or bone metastases or nearing the end of an opioid dose, although the cause is often unknown. Most of the time, this pain is short term, lasting less than thirty minutes, but it can happen several times a day, and it can be difficult to treat because it's unpredictable. Perhaps it was this kind of breakthrough pain that caused my mother's severe episode, and what she endured couldn't have been foreseen or prevented.

UNCONSCIOUS PAIN

Still another type of pain that can be difficult to treat is pain that's hard for physicians to see, like the pain that unconscious patients sometimes experience.

Like most dying people, my mother spent her last few days either sleeping or only semiconscious. She didn't cry out or moan, except during that one excruciating episode. My best guess would be that she was not in significant pain most of the time, but I don't know that for certain.

Just because patients are unconscious doesn't mean they don't feel pain, says Céline Gélinas, an associate professor at McGill University's school of nursing. "There's no clear evidence that they cannot feel pain," she says. She recounts a decades-old study in which patients who survived cardiac arrests were asked to describe their physical experiences. "Some of them even remembered the pain from the defibrillation," Gélinas says. "So, we cannot conclude that [unconscious patients] do not feel pain at all. It's still possible."

When Gélinas first began working as a nurse, she was frustrated that some physicians were unwilling to treat pain in unconscious patients. "At the time, we had no tool to assess pain in patients unable to self-report," she says. So Gélinas returned to graduate school where she helped develop the Critical-Care Pain Observation Tool, an assessment based on precise analysis of patients' facial expressions, body movements, muscle tension, and vocalizations—whether patients are crying out or moaning.

People who are in pain look distressed—even when they are unconscious, they often make a face, says Margaret Campbell, the professor of nursing at Wayne State University. "You can walk into a room—anybody can walk into a room—and see when someone is upset," she says. "We know when something is wrong with another person, including physical changes, if we're good at looking at faces and looking at body language."

On the other hand, if a dying patient is lying completely still in bed, with a relaxed face and no muscle tension, perhaps with a partially opened mouth and eyes, a careful observer knows the patient isn't in pain, she says. "That person is so comfortable, they're not even blinking or closing their mouth."

Both Campbell and Gélinas have studied those kinds of expressions and signs in detail. For instance, Gélinas explains that facial expressions that express fear are very different from those that express pain: People's eyebrows usually rise up when they're afraid, and their eyes will open more widely. When they're in pain, their eyebrows tend to go down and their eyes close. She's tested her observations and created a scale so that physicians will have a better idea of when to treat pain for unconscious patients.

Emery Brown, a neuroscientist and a professor of anesthesia at Harvard Medical School, analyzes pain in unconscious patients from another angle. Because unconsciousness in anesthetized patients is controlled, patients' states can be carefully monitored. And anesthesiologists are very aware that their patients may be unconscious and unable to perceive pain, and yet be affected by it. "We see this all the time under anesthesia," Brown says. "It's very, very real." Anesthesiologists can recognize the effects of this pain because they typically monitor blood pressure, heart rate, and oxygen levels in patients undergoing surgery.

"Let's just say I gave you drugs which made you unconscious, and then I let the surgeons perform surgery on you and I didn't give you anything that would block your pain pathways," Brown says. "I could tell that you were in pain from what they were doing, because I might see your heart rate and blood pressure go up. In other words, the systems that process pain are still active. But your consciousness is turned off, and [yet] it's very clear to me you're perceiving pain."

These patients are always given other medications to treat this physical pain, he says. "You have to, because if you don't they'll have a heart attack right there in front of you." The body's pain receptors are activating, and stress systems are responding.

In dying people, unlike most patients under anesthesia, the brain eventually breaks down so far that they are no longer capable of consciously registering pain. The problem is that it's not easy to identify exactly when this happens.

That means it's hard to know for certain how much patients are suffering. "However, we generally believe that if your brain is really in a comatose kind of situation, or you're not really responsive, that your perception—how you feel about things—may also be significantly decreased," says David Hui, an oncologist and palliative care specialist who researches the signs of approaching death. "You may or may not even be aware of what's happening."

PALLIATIVE SEDATION

In a few rare cases, Hallenbeck says, pain in dying people can be very difficult or impossible to control. Sometimes, moving patients to a residential hospice or hospital allows doctors more options for effective treatment. Sometimes, more highly skilled palliative care doctors can get the pain under control. "There can be cases where specialists really help," Hallenbeck says. They can rapidly titrate drugs to bring someone's extreme pain down out of the stratosphere. "The average doc's not going to know that kind of stuff."

There are also rare cases in which a dying patient's suffering can't be relieved with typical drugs. Doctors will then sometimes give patients a sedative so heavy it basically conks them out. This is called palliative sedation therapy, and it's still relatively controversial, mostly because people confuse it with euthanasia. Palliative sedation is different, however. It involves using drugs to keep patients unconscious to ease their pain—not to shorten their lives. And this method doesn't usually mean sedating patients deeply and continuously until their deaths. Patients are more often given repeated doses of medicine, usually small enough to allow doctors to communicate with them from time to time.

Still, even people who have a good grasp on the distinction between palliative sedation and euthanasia sometimes feel uneasy about sedating dying patients. "To intentionally reduce patient awareness, even consensually, is a decision requiring careful consideration," cautions a paper based on research by a panel of international palliative care experts. "Sedation may mean that completing the tasks of life's end are short-circuited or prevented." If patients are sedated to the point of unconsciousness in their last days, they can't say final good-byes, can't ask or grant forgiveness for old feuds, can't reexamine their lives for meaning.

Because palliative sedation means intentionally taking away the possibility of awareness so close to death and because of societal fears that it might hasten death, it is rarely used. Instead, most dying patients drift more and more deeply into unconsciousness simply because their bodies, including their brains, are shutting down.

SO, *DOES* DYING HURT OR DOESN'T IT? AND WHY?

In hindsight, there might have been several reasons for my mother's extreme pain in her last few days. It might have been breakthrough pain, perhaps the result of organs in her system breaking down or metastases to her bones. Because that kind of pain is so random, it's difficult to foresee. As someone dying with metastasized breast cancer, my mother was receiving the typical treatment of regular, "by-the-clock" doses of opioids for continual pain with extra medication on hand to treat breakthrough pain. But because she was unconscious, it would have been hard for anyone to realize the pain was building. She was given extra medication after she was in convulsions, but then it took time to get the pain back under control.

It's also possible she hadn't swallowed her last dose of morphine—that it had trickled down her chin and no one noticed, although I think that's unlikely. I believe there's even a chance that she wasn't actually feeling pain: While her body responded as if she were suffering terribly, it's conceivable that she was not.

Most of the hospice patients I've watched have wrestled with pain or discomfort at some point. In the two most difficult cases, the patients moaned or called out as nurses worked frantically to control their pain. I've sat with other patients as they've labored to cough or just breathe, and now and then, a patient's constipation or nausea has seemed excruciating for two or three hours.

But in each of the cases I've witnessed, the pain and discomfort were temporary. A problem surfaced, nurses worked with patients to address it, and it was at least managed or controlled. By the time the patients died, they seemed peaceful.

The bottom line is that dying people don't have to experience significant pain, writes Holly Prigerson, director of the Center for Research on End of Life Care at Cornell. "Patients do not need to die in pain if they have adequate opioids and other medications."

Saunders felt she could relieve most—though not all—of her dying patients' pain: "I do not claim that none of my patients suffer any pain or distress at all, but only that I try and keep it within their own personal limits of endurance," she writes.

> She said, "It doesn't hurt—I thought it would hurt."
> I said, "What doesn't hurt?"
> I was wondering if something was wrong with her arm, her leg, her hip—and she said, "Dying—it doesn't hurt." —HOSPICE NURSE

Researchers have found that dying patients often fear pain more than they fear death itself. Hallenbeck says it's understandable that people are afraid of pain and other physical symptoms associated with dying. "With a competent team, I do not fear physical pain at the end of life," he told me. "For the physical stuff I'm pretty optimistic for myself and for others that with good care—which we're still working hard to get in a lot of places—things aren't bad."

He added this: "Which begs the question, then, what *am* I afraid of?"

So, I asked him.

"Most of the suffering that I see toward the end of life is from people's unresolved issues in their life," he said. He gave the example of his parents, both of whom were doctors. They had different, rare forms of dementia at the end of life. His mother had Lewy body dementia, and his father's dementia seemed to have been influenced by the polio he'd contracted earlier in life.

But something other than the physical diseases caused the greatest suffering for both of them as they died, he says. "My mother was particularly attached to being Dr. Hallenbeck," he explains. "She had to have it on her nursing home room door, and I saw how much suffering holding on to that caused her." Neither of his parents coped well with dying, and that caused them greater suffering, he says.

And in both cases, he feels they could have done something to prevent it.

chapter six
coping: a map for how to die well

WHEN MY MOTHER suddenly couldn't keep track of how many pills she'd taken, or whether she'd taken any pills—oxycodone for pain and other medications to treat the oxycodone's side effects—my family realized she wasn't her old self, that in fact, she was rapidly approaching death. We moved into my parents' house: my husband and I, my brother, his wife, and sometimes their two children. My sister and her boyfriend flew in from Reno. My mother's two brothers and a sister-in-law traveled from Illinois and kept vigil with us for two nights.

We slipped into our roles as if we'd been tending to the dying all our lives. We took turns cooking and sitting by my mother's bedside as she floated in and out of consciousness, telling each other stories, laughing, giggling, crying. We grocery-shopped for large numbers of people. We gathered in the living room to listen as my father played the piano—old Broadway tunes, hymns, folk songs, and Beethoven sonatas, my mother smiling from where she lay on the couch.

She did still smile, hold our hands, and talk a little, and there were times when she sparkled with some of her old energy, but with each day, she was unconscious or asleep for longer periods. My mother was not fully present; she couldn't be.

But we were. We'd always been a close family, with my mother at our center. This was different. When we were around her now we felt a peace, a dropping-away of all the unimportant things. Time was filled with something other people wanted to be part of—a friend called it "sacredness." Visitors lingered, trying to soak it in. My family felt especially connected with each other; we felt a fresh awareness of life's beauty and brevity; we felt grateful for whatever time we still had with my mother; we simply *felt*, profoundly, in ways we never had before.

When Ira Byock, the physician who writes about dying, cared for his dying father, he also found the experience difficult but deeply meaningful. He writes that it transformed his understanding of what dying meant—or, at least, what it might mean. After his father's death, Byock began to observe his dying patients and their caregivers more closely. He noticed that a few of their experiences were rich and rewarding in the way his own family's had been:

> Every once in a while a family would return after a
> patient died and say that their loved one's passing
> had been extraordinary. "When we heard Mama was
> terminal, it was the worst thing that ever happened to
> our family, but this last month with her was some of the
> best time we have ever spent together" was the sort of
> comment I had occasionally heard before but had always
> dismissed as a peculiar, if pleasant, phenomenon.

For the first time, Byock realized that while good deaths might be uncommon, they were real. As he continued to talk with dying patients and their caregivers, he had a second revelation: "good deaths were not random events or matters of luck; they could be understood and, perhaps, fostered."

WHAT IS A GOOD DEATH?

"People die the way they've lived," hospice professionals will say, shaking their heads at the emotional drama surrounding many dying patients—the way some patients lash out at nurses simply for being unfamiliar, or for breaking a glass, or for nothing; the arguments between exes and current spouses about who's allowed at the bedside; the disagreements between friends and family members about medications or treatment plans.

But the kinds of peaceful deaths Byock and I both witnessed are not unique. When Avery Weisman and J. William Worden did their classic study of newly diagnosed cancer patients, they found that "many patients seem to cope effectively with their plight, participating fully in treatment and, in general, refuting the expectation of inevitable alarm and inexorable disaster." And anyone who works with dying people seems to have a story about how, occasionally, a patient with a fatal condition emanates a greater sense of vitality, or peace and wisdom, or even joy, than anyone else.

An emergency room technician once telephoned James Hallenbeck, the palliative care expert who is also a hospice doctor, to tell him about an eighty-five-year-old man who, although he had no major symptoms, claimed he was dying. "He's perfectly fine with that," the tech told Hallenbeck, "but he didn't want to disturb anybody by someone finding his body somewhere. So he wondered if we had a spot where he could go and do this thing."

When Hallenbeck met with him, the man struck him as rational, calm, and at peace with what he saw as his imminent death. He reminisced about his many close friends and family, all of whom were now dead. He talked about the fulfilling jobs he'd held as an antiques restorer and amateur musician. He told Hallenbeck he didn't know how he knew, but he was sure that he was now dying. Hallenbeck believed the man's self-diagnosis:

So I said, "Is there anything I can do for you?" I was almost in tears by this point; I was blown away by this guy's life story and the level of acceptance. It was like Zen masters who used to call people in and say, "I'm passing away and here's my poem," and then died sitting in Zazen . . . He said, "Yeah, you know, I can't get this remote control to work and I always watch Jeopardy at seven thirty." . . . I said, "I think we can help you with that."

Hallenbeck had someone fix the remote control, and he also wrote a prescription for an antianxiety drug, which the man never took. He died that night.

The man's calm acceptance of death made a lasting impression on Hallenbeck, who views it as something to aspire to. "I don't think I'll ever get that close, but I know in my bones that it's possible," he says.

Cicely Saunders, the British hospice pioneer, also had patients who coped especially well with their approaching deaths. One of her most memorable patients was "Mrs. G," a young woman whose disease left her gradually more and more paralyzed and blind until, in her last three years, she lost her sight completely and she could barely move at all. Despite her physical hardships, the woman was a sunny presence on the ward, popular among staff members and other patients. Saunders writes that after spending time at her bedside one afternoon, another patient said, "The incredible thing is, you don't even feel sorry for her; she is so alive." The young woman's attitude toward death had an enduring impact on Saunders and the rest of the medical staff. With Mrs. G in mind, Saunders would later write, "Many of us can look back and say firmly of those we have lost, however hard and lonely their path may have seemed, that it is not what dying did to them that we remember, but what they have done to our thoughts on death."

My mother's experience and those of the dying patients Hallenbeck and Saunders describe were significantly different from each other. My mother was surrounded by family and friends at home when she died, while Hallenbeck's patient was singularly alone. And in contrast to both of them, Saunders's patient suffered from debilitating side effects of her disease for years. Yet all three had "good deaths"—a reminder of why palliative care experts often caution against using the term. It can sound prescriptive, as if there's one right way, or as if all of us should want exactly the same kind of death. The idea of a certain kind of good death can also ignore the way values change and people adapt as we near the end of life.

But most dying people do seem to share the same general desires, says Gary Rodin, the palliative care specialist trained in both internal medicine and psychiatry. Those desires are fairly consistent across cultures, although people's specific expectations of how those needs are met vary a lot, depending on where they live or what resources they have. "The things people want at the end of life, no matter where you are, are not very different," Rodin says. "People want relief from suffering, people want to die in the location of [their] choice, and they want to have a sense of closure on their life, a sense that their life was meaningful. They want people who are important [to them] to be with them."

If we know we're dying, what we want—in general—is pretty universal. And based on the experiences of some dying patients, we know it's at least possible to die well. The question remains: How do we get there? If dying is a journey, surely there must be some kind of map.

"NO ONE IN THE BIBLE DIED LIKE THIS"

Guidance for dying people was once widely available through churches and cultural traditions. When a relative was dying, you called the priest or minister and he could steer you through the ceremonies and duties required of the living. Or you might turn to neighbors for help in caring for the dying. Religious institutions and texts oversaw the process, and health care services played only a small role.

Now medical systems allow many people to accumulate diseases, any one of which would have killed them in the past. At the same time, the system fails to provide enough support in other ways, and patients often feel lost. "As a patient once told me, 'No one in the Bible died like this,'" writes Joanne Lynn, the hospice physician and palliative care advocate. "People find little guidance when they look to our ancient texts for comfort and advice on how to live while walking a tightrope of serious illness and frailty, propped up by modern medicine."

As a result, people diagnosed with fatal diseases often feel "essentially untaught and unpracticed," writes the nurse researcher Nessa Coyle. When Coyle conducted a series of indepth interviews with seven advanced-cancer patients—six of whom would die by the end of her study—the patients told her they felt unprepared for the tasks associated with dying: "We all don't know—how does one die? Nobody teaches you."

If you're diagnosed with a terminal disease, the set of problems you'll face is fairly predictable, Rodin says. But, like other palliative care researchers, Rodin was initially struck by the fact that "in spite of how predictable the problems are, there hasn't been an organized approach to help people with those problems."

That's starting to change.

COPING STRATEGIES

In their study, Weisman and Worden tried to predict which patients would cope best with their disease. Patients were asked what disease-associated problems they were facing, what cop-

ing strategies they were using, and what the results were in re-
solving the problems. While the researchers acknowledge that
it's impossible to list every possible coping method, they developed a list of fifteen general techniques used by patients. The
techniques, which ranged from confronting issues directly, to
researching, to talking through problems with others, weren't
always effective, and much depended on a patient's social or
emotional condition.

"Not every strategy can be used by everyone," Weisman and
Worden caution, and different problems call for different solutions. Some patients were more vulnerable than others because of their family or social situations. But they found that
the good copers—those who were less emotionally or socially
vulnerable and were able to resolve many of their issues—
tended to "face facts, find something favorable, and then
confidently comply with the doctor's recommendations." In
contrast, poor copers tended to "refuse to acknowledge more
than a minimum about illness, talk very little, and either ca-
pitulate passively or inappropriately act out."

Some coping strategies that seemed on the surface to be
good solutions weren't very successful. For instance, seeking
out more information and sharing your concerns with other
people seem like obviously good coping strategies, but in the
study, these strategies were often ineffective for patients. The
researchers theorize that the strategies tend to be effective
when they're actually used to cope with a diagnosis, but they
don't work well when they're used as ways to avoid the problem: "For example, patients can seek more information only
to question the facts and continue the search for a more ac-
ceptable answer," they write. "They may share worries with
others, but only to have a handy sounding board for the question, Why me?"

While Weisman and Worden's study is still influential, it's
now decades old. Since then, psychologists, social workers, and

medical professionals have begun researching techniques—psychologists call them "interventions"—to help people cope better with dying. Some of those interventions have been tested in randomized, controlled trials, and they've been found to make a significant difference. The interventions share similar features. Typically, they consist of sessions with a trained professional in which patients discuss their own mortality, their feelings about a difficult diagnosis, their grief. The clinician guides them in a life review, and then tries to help them re-create a sense of meaning. Perhaps most importantly, the interventions help patients create space and time to think.

Byock, Rodin, and Virginia Lee, the nurse researcher, are part of a growing number of experts who are developing coping methods and publishing research about them. Through studies and patient interviews, they're creating an array of maps for dying people: ways for patients to navigate the process better in modern societies. Ways to die well.

WHAT'S THE MEANING OF LIFE IF YOU'RE DYING?

When Lee began her career as a nurse at a bone marrow transplantation unit, many of the patients she saw were either on the brink of dying or—if the transplants worked—experiencing a kind of rebirth. While most of them struggled with extreme uncertainty just after their diagnosis, a few did "fantastically well," she says. Lee, who also has a degree in psychology, wondered why. So she began interviewing patients about how they were coping, and she discovered that one of the main problems for people diagnosed with serious illnesses is that they lose the sense that their lives are meaningful. For many people, that loss means that their world falls apart.

Some of Lee's patients, however, seemed more resilient. They came up with a new sense of meaning that fit their changed lives, and that was true whether they were newly diagnosed, in the middle of treatment, or dying from their disease. In one of the exercises Lee has her patients do, she asks them to draw a line representing their lives, and then place a circle where they think they are along that line—near the end? At the beginning or middle?

No matter what their age or diagnosis, most people place the circle about three-quarters of the way along the line; they see their lives as roughly three-quarters over. But not everyone, she says. She was surprised to see that some patients—not many—drew the circle at the very beginning of their line. "It was incredible," Lee says. "These are patients that immediately told me that they've gone through all this reflection; they know what their priorities are." For these patients, a diagnosis with a serious disease felt like a wake-up call that placed them at the start of a new life. "They thought it was their second chance to really live meaningfully."

Lee, who is now an assistant professor of nursing at McGill University, was particularly impressed when young people discovered a sense of renewed meaning through their cancer diagnosis. "Some of them—not a lot, but maybe one or two—would come up and say, 'This is the best thing that happened because now I know what I want to do with my life,'" she says. They'd tell her, "I'm not going to waste my time anymore."

The resilience Lee was seeing in some of her patients is a primary human motivation. Everyone has it to some degree, but sometimes, people need outside help to stimulate that innate resilience, she explains. So Lee took what she learned from her interviews with people who were coping well, and "kind of bottled all of that up into one intervention." She has used the intervention to help patients with different types and stages of cancer; some have a realistic chance at recovery, others eventually die from their disease. In a pilot study, for instance, Lee offered the intervention to women diagnosed with advanced ovarian cancer. For most of these patients, the odds of surviving five years are usually less than 50 percent. Lee now focuses on newly diagnosed patients because, she emphasizes, even if they have a fatal disease, "they have so much living ahead of them."

In the intervention, patients meet with a trained oncologist or psychotherapist—in her original study, this was Lee. The clinician helps patients re-create meaning by encouraging them to review their lives, to face the sorts of questions they are often already asking themselves:

Did my life have meaning?
Did I contribute something?
What am I leaving to my children, or to my colleagues
at work if I don't have children, or to my spouse, to my
friends?
Did my existence make any difference in the world?
Because I know now that I am about to leave this world,
was it all for naught, or what impact, what value did it
have?

In four sessions, patients are guided through a series of storytelling tasks to reflect on their cancer and its implications for them.

In the first session, patients discuss what's happening to them in the present—their diagnosis with a serious disease, their feelings about the diagnosis, their grief. "I acknowledge that it is a really bad time," Lee says, "like, maybe the worst time of their life that they are coping with right now."

But then while I'm listening to all that, as they're
telling their story, I'm looking for areas in their life that
they can still control, that are not so bad, that they can

still find pleasure in, that they still have meaningful moments in. And I reflect that back to them. So I'm giving them a balanced life view now with cancer.

The second task involves reflecting on past challenges. "I build the sense of resilience by looking back at other life events that were as unexpected as cancer—maybe not to the same magnitude—but they were unexpected, uncontrollable, unpredictable," she says. Jobs or promotions they didn't receive, sometimes through no fault of their own. Partners who had affairs, or relationships that soured or ended. Serious falls, car crashes, other diseases.

Lee asks patients how they coped with those past challenges, reminding them that they have the capacity to apply the same approach with cancer.

In the third task, patients talk about the future: about their priorities and goals "within the context of an acknowledged mortality."

Lee did a clinical trial with seventy-four patients who had colorectal or breast cancer, half of whom received the intervention and half of whom did not, although members of the control group were free to seek other psychological support, just as ordinary patients would be. Patients' responses to the intervention were powerful, she says. Those who received the intervention all emerged with an improved sense of themselves or their self-esteem. "They felt more optimistic about the future, even though they have cancer, and they all improved in their sense of self-efficacy."

Lee has watched patients develop a better sense of resilience through the intervention, and she's observed that they also develop "a greater sense of compassion for other people." Her concern now is getting the intervention to more patients. She has created a workbook that guides people through the series of reflection exercises on their own, and she's also working on an app.

A COUPLE OF CAVEATS

Lee learned the hard way that it's crucial not to imply that patients should be relentlessly positive. When she was piloting her intervention, her first patient said she was struggling with her diagnosis: "I can't go up this flight of stairs, and I read all these books about how people are doing so well," the patient told Lee. "I feel so bad about myself; I feel even worse because I'm not like everyone else."

"Thank God it was the first intervention," Lee says, "because then I switched the way that I introduced the intervention. What's important for me, that I stress to my students, is that patients need to know that they have that chance to grieve and look at the changes and the losses in their lives."

Lee and other palliative care experts caution that being diagnosed with a serious or fatal disease is always difficult. "Skeptics of the idea of dying well like to remind me that death is hardly beautiful and is often messy and unpleasant," Byock writes in his book, *Dying Well.* "And I readily agree. Even for people who do die well, the process of dying is rarely enjoyable; indeed, it is commonly a wrenching time in one's life."

For some, even the terms *good death* or *dying well* are troubling not only because of the prescriptive implications but also because the terms suggest that patients have an obligation to cope well—at the same time they're struggling with pain and loss and suffering. Dying patients in a study conducted by nursing researcher Judith Wrubel told her about the pressure they felt to be upbeat: "no matter how positive an attitude one has, or how much one embraces the moment, there remains the daily reality of illness, symptoms and suffering," she summarizes. "There is no 'good' way to cope that will make those things go away." Furthermore, it's unfair to expect dying people to fulfill superhuman roles, Wrubel writes. Many people with terminal diseases rise to the occasion, facing their condition with courage that seems impossibly heroic to others. We often place these people on pedestals. But that can mask the hardships they actually live, the real ways they're affected by disease, and the way their lives continue to have both peaks and valleys. Even people who deal exceptionally well with their diagnoses express anger and frustration or exhaustion at times.

Dying usually means facing harder challenges than you've faced at any other time in life. Coping skills and interventions can help. But palliative care specialist Gary Rodin says it's important to remember that "there's a suffering that can't be eliminated."

CALM

When Rodin and his colleagues at the Princess Margaret Cancer Centre in Toronto conducted a study of their advanced cancer patients' emotional states, they found that at any one time, a quarter of them had significant symptoms of depression and hopelessness. So Rodin's team decided to do something. They began interviewing patients about the issues they were facing, and from those conversations, they developed an intervention of their own.

They found that patients were often overwhelmed by dealing with medical treatments, which meant they had little time or energy to devote to *living* in their remaining months or years. "The main problem is to be able to think about dying and to continue living—that's what our intervention is trying to help people do," Rodin says.

Rodin and his colleagues knew that patients needed time

and space set aside for reflection, and the patients would benefit from working with trained professionals. They wanted to create semi-structured sessions so patients would receive guidance in thinking through the complexity of issues they were facing, but would also have some leeway to deal with whatever issues were most pressing.

Rodin's team named their intervention "CALM," which stands for "[Managing] Cancer and Living Meaningfully." The technique itself is relatively simple: Over the course of a few months, patients meet with a trained mental health professional for six sessions of about an hour each. The therapist guides them through discussions covering four general domains, but patients get to decide whether to focus on multiple domains at once, how much time to spend in each, or even which domains to cover in each session. While the domains are numbered for ease of reference, patients can choose to delve into the second or third or fourth domain first, or cover two domains in a single session, or change the order of the domains in other ways.

The first domain focuses on pragmatic health issues. In this domain, Rodin says, patients and therapists address questions such as, "How do you manage your symptoms? How do you talk to your doctors? How do you make a decision about clinical trials? All those things about your relationship with the health care system, which becomes extremely important."

If you're diagnosed with a serious disease, chances are it may be the first time you've come up against the complexity of modern medical systems, Rodin says. Oncology visits tend to be brief and focused and patients often don't have a chance to explore in depth the information and options they're finding out from doctors. In contrast, the CALM intervention gives patients an opportunity to discuss what's going on. A patient's wife told Rodin's team that the therapy sessions were the first time she and her husband, who had been seen by several different specialists, felt they were being treated as full human beings by the medical system. "Everybody kind of looks at him as: 'there's a lung problem and there's a bone problem, and there's a skin problem,' so everybody is solving these little problems and nobody is looking at him as a person," she told the researchers.

CALM therapists also encourage patients to avoid allowing medical issues to take over their lives, Rodin says. "There's kind of an illusion that there'll be some later time to live your life—which there isn't," he says. "You need to be able to live your life at the same time." When you have a terminal disease, it's easy for your disease and the medical system to take over your life. You often have to make difficult decisions about what kind of treatment to pursue, whether to participate in clinical trials, and whether to continue treatments at all. It's tempting to spend all your time researching the best possible treatments, even after what's available becomes less and less effective. If you have the money, there are always more doctors with experimental techniques, more clinics where you can travel for new treatment methods, more drugs or surgeries you can try.

But rather than allowing a disheartening quest for more treatments to steal your remaining time, you need to learn what and how to ask doctors about delicate subjects, Rodin says. Questions about the evidence that a particular therapy will add significant time to your life, about whether you're really a good treatment candidate, about the quality of life you might expect and which treatments might add or take away from that quality. If you don't find a way to bring up those questions, you may find yourself continuing with a treatment plan that doesn't match your wishes.

Rodin has heard the treatment process compared to a train: Doctors start patients on a treatment plan, and once it gets going, round after round of chemotherapy drugs or other protocols are prescribed almost automatically. At worst, treatments that are painful and debilitating continue even when they won't alleviate difficult symptoms or lengthen a patient's life span: "It's easier for the train to keep moving, the treatments just to keep being prescribed," Rodin says, rather than stopping to discuss whether each decision makes sense for particular patients at particular points in their disease progression.

The answer isn't always clear; sometimes, chemotherapy or radiation is used to reduce painful tumors; sometimes, patients are willing to suffer a great deal in order to extend their lives even for a few extra weeks. Rodin says he and other therapists don't try to give advice on whether or not to continue treatment, but they do try to help patients understand the implications of making particular choices.

The second domain in Rodin's intervention focuses on the drastic changes in a person's sense of identity and relationships that can happen when someone is diagnosed with a serious disease. "Everything that makes you feel good about yourself—the way you look, your physical appearance, your physical function, your ability to work and engage in family and social relations—all those things get undermined by a cancer like this," Rodin says. That can also happen with relationships. "You might need something different from your relationships." Perhaps you've been a caretaker for children or elderly parents, but now you'll be the one who's dependent.

Patients tell Rodin and his colleagues that simply having a chance to talk with therapists about the differences in how other people interact with them helps. One patient noted that cancer was "recalibrating" the patient's relationships with friends. "There are people who desperately want to be part of this because they want to help," the patient told the researchers. "And there are people who are very uncomfortable with this and don't even want to talk about it and then there are people that may want to help but I actually don't want them to help." The therapy allowed the patient to simply let other people be themselves, rather than judging them based on their reactions to the disease.

A family member or caregiver is encouraged to come for at least one of the six sessions in the intervention, and the joint sessions help patients and caregivers support each other. "Just about in every one of these cases, to be diagnosed in this way is a personal and family catastrophe," Rodin says. "And the catastrophe's affecting not only the patient but the family."

In fact, spouses are sometimes more distressed than patients. "When you come closer to the end of life, your frame gets narrower; there's not as many worries," he says. In contrast, family members tend to have even more concerns than usual. At some point, patients are no longer engaged in the day-to-day practicalities like grocery shopping, preparing meals, paying bills, or organizing care for themselves. At some point, the patient usually stops thinking about longer-term financial issues, "whereas the spouse has to think about not only the present but also the future in a different way," Rodin says. The joint sessions allow patients and caregivers a place to talk about those concerns in a way that feels safe—that won't endanger their relationships or feel hurtful.

The third domain focuses on therapists' guiding patients in seeking a renewed sense of meaning and spiritual well-being. After the first existential shock of learning they have a fatal disease, Rodin says, people begin to look more deeply at how a terminal diagnosis changes the meaning of their lives. Not surprisingly, there's a sense of urgency in the search for meaning for patients with a fatal disease. "We all should be thinking about this—which is maybe the value in being involved with patients like this—but people who have a year to live, or something like that, *have* to think about what's important in their life," Rodin points out. "People need to sort of re-find their own sense of meaning, their own value in themselves."

The fourth domain focuses on mortality. Whether or not patients are religious, they usually want to address changed priorities and existential questions, Rodin says. And this can help them both in very down-to-earth ways such as creating living wills and doing advanced care planning, and also in more metaphysical ways, such as coming to terms with fears about dying.

The researchers say patients often feel there's an "unspoken taboo about raising the topic of death and dying with friends and family, although this issue was what often concerned them the most." In the CALM sessions, they felt free to explore questions about their own mortality: to talk about what they thought would happen to them after they died, about their fears about suffering, or even about the fact that they *weren't* afraid. Patients expressed great relief simply at having the topic of death broached with a therapist. And after discussing their feelings about dying with the CALM therapist, they were sometimes ready to discuss the subject with family or friends.

After participating in a CALM study, patients have reported they like the mix of practical and emotional/spiritual assistance—addressing both questions about how to manage symptoms as well as whether to participate in clinical trials or continue a treatment, Rodin says. Based on qualitative data, "we have no doubt that it's enormously helpful to people."

For those who don't have access to a therapist or interventions like CALM, there are still models for learning to cope better with dying. One of those is Byock's "four things that matter most"—which is also the title of his book.

FOUR THINGS THAT MATTER: A DIY MODEL

Byock says he's not sure exactly how he came up with his list of four statements that dying people should say to the people they love. Long ago, he remembers listening as a social worker or nurse in Fresno helped dying patients find some sort of resolution in their lives. He built on the advice she offered, and he recalls asking patients in his early clinical work a question he still raises:

> "If, heaven forbid, you or someone you love were to die suddenly, as any of us might, would there be important things that you would feel would be left unsaid between you and someone you love"—sometimes I ask, "or *once loved*"—"like a previous husband or wife?"
>
> Not uncommonly, when I pose that question, and I pose it in a kind of wondering aloud kind of tone, people will look at me as if I've just read their mind, as if, "How did you know?"
>
> And I'll say, "Well, you know, it's common. It turns out, we matter a lot to one another."

Humans are hard-wired in a way that makes other humans much more important to us than things or activities, Byock says. And because of that, dying people need a sense of completion with the people who have mattered most to them in their lives. Completing relationships isn't the same as ending them: Survivors continue to have a relationship with people who have died—the relationship doesn't end with death. But it's complete when you've said everything important you need to say to each other.

For example, Byock says he feels that kind of completion with his father, and their relationship is still very much alive despite his father's death: "I wouldn't say I talk to him exactly, but he's certainly in my mind as I observe certain things, or go through certain experiences, and kind of wish he was there to talk with or share."

The guidelines Byock provides for achieving a sense of completion are a set of four succinct statements for dying people to say to their loved ones, statements distilled from the issues he has discussed with patients over the years:

Please forgive me.
I forgive you.
Thank you.
I love you.

And, he adds: Good-bye.

In *Dying Well* and *The Four Things That Matter Most,* Byock has described some of the situations in which he's witnessed the effectiveness of the four statements, and the ways that saying them have led dying people to find meaning and peace. They can help both dying people and their family members heal old wounds. Even in good relationships, the statements often make a difference, he writes. They allow families a way to talk about their grief with each other and to share happy memories.

Once patients begin to think about these four topics, they sometimes realize there are other valuable things they need to say to their family. He told me about an interview with a woman who had metastatic cancer:

She said, "My daughter's never found herself; she's actually successful, but she's a single mom and she's never had luck with men, and she's seeing this shrink in Boston," and she rolled her eyes, you know, "Two hundred dollars an hour, twice a week," and as I listened to her and let her talk, I was just sort of leaning forward and listening closely.

After she was done, I said, "You know, it occurs to me, you clearly love your children, and I don't want to be presumptuous, but if you could find even one thing to say to each of them, to say not only the four things we've talked about, but to express your love and then to say, 'You know, I'm proud of you; I'm proud to be your mom,' what a gift that would be. I mean, who else on the planet could give that gift?"

The woman began to cry, Byock told me. "I was just breathing and just letting it unfold—very centered—and then she started to giggle. And that sort of drew me off center, and I said, 'Tell me, why are you laughing? What's up?'"

The woman replied, "Well, that's what she needs, Dr. Byock. She needs her mother to tell her how much I love her and how proud I am." Then both Byock and the mother started laughing at how simple their realization seemed, and yet how crucial it was. Byock says that if he were to add another thing to his book's list of the four things that matter, it would probably be "I'm proud of you"—especially for parents to say to their children.

Byock returns to one point over and over: that dying people still have something to contribute to their loved ones and to the community. The rest of society often forgets this. A terminal diagnosis is too often understood to mean that life is over, or, at least, the chance for meaningful life. People too often believe that terminally ill patients have nothing left to give back to society. That hasn't been Byock's experience.

MAYBE IT HELPS TO GET TO WORK EARLIER

After Hallenbeck watched his parents suffer through holding on so tightly to their old identities when they were dying, he promised himself he'd try to avoid that self-inflicted suffering. So he's practicing letting go now. "I think the work that people need to do, to suffer less in dying, paradoxically, more often than not, has to be done before they die," he says. He contrasts two dying patients, both with similar levels of dementia, who were having their diapers changed. One was mortified by the experience, and Hallenbeck remembers him saying some version of the following: "Oh, the indignity of it all—how could this happen to me? It's so undignified." The other expressed only gratitude to the nurse's aide: "Thank you, honey, thank you so much for doing this. I'm so grateful that you are changing this diaper for me."

Despite the similar circumstances, one patient was suffering much more than the other. The people who tend to suffer less, Hallenbeck believes, have examined their lives deeply and tried to make important changes *before* they're dying. "The ones that are really holding on to something, and they can't let it go, or some great regret—they suffer the most, and we don't have an easy pill for that."

PEACEFUL DYING

Still, even in the last weeks or days of life, people sometimes find peace or bring a sense of meaning and grace to those around them.

That was true for my mother, who was under hospice care at home. Dad had sent word to their friends in Kentucky, where they lived for more than forty years, that Mom was dying and now the letters and e-mails began to arrive. One of us would read them aloud to Mom, and then read them again, because she had fallen asleep.

"I like the sound of your voices," Mom said. She seemed unaffected by the praises heaped upon her, the tributes and compliments from people I had forgotten or never heard of—people who said she had been like a second mother to them, that she had been a light of intellect, that she was the one person they felt they could talk to, confide in.

When we finished reading letters to her, we read poetry.

We read William Wordsworth, Robert Service and Walt Whitman, Emily Dickinson and Wendell Berry and Mary Oliver. My brother's children sometimes read, too, their tongues stumbling over the nineteenth-century diction. The same poems kept getting repeated, but no one minded.

One afternoon, a childhood friend and I sat on the carpeted floor and sang songs from when we were little: the folk song, "Ho, Young Rider, Apple-cheeked One, Whither Riding?" and "Try Not to Get Worried," from *Jesus Christ Superstar*. We kept our untrained voices soft. Mom was asleep, or maybe in far-off daydreams. We felt again like little girls, sitting in the corner of the room holding hands, our eyes distracted with memories.

Her eyes had closed again but she smiled, and settled slightly, waiting.

chapter seven
growth and legacies

PEOPLE WHO ARE DIAGNOSED with a fatal disease sometimes do more than cope. They grow. They repair or strengthen relationships. They find a deeper spirituality or meaning in the life that remains for them. They create a legacy of good memories for the people they leave behind. When any of this happens, it tends to happen *because of*—not *despite*—the challenges of facing death and struggling with pain and loss.

Before she became a hospice nurse, Deb Callahan was a neonatal nurse. While she loved working with premature babies, witnessing their difficulties underlined for her the importance of time in the womb. "Babies need that forty weeks of gestation, to be forming and developing," she says. Callahan, who is now a hospice volunteer, believes something similar is true at the other end of the spectrum, in the last few weeks of dying from a terminal disease. "A lot of things happen in those weeks, especially with relationships," she says. She has watched at the bedsides of dying people as some have mended family relationships or brought a sense of deeper meaning and joy to those around them. And when her mother was diagnosed with a fatal disease, Callahan observed her growing and developing as she faced death: "My mom was kind of a fearful person," Callahan remembers. "It was just amazing to me how she transformed after getting the terminal diagnosis."

"Mrs. G," the young mother whom hospice pioneer Cicely Saunders describes as one of her most memorable patients, suffered not only from blindness and paralysis, but several severe setbacks—her legs had to be strapped down during the day or they jerked, and during her last two and a half years, those muscle spasms became very painful. But in the midst of her drawn-out dying, Mrs. G was "triumphant," Saunders writes. She influenced hundreds of people: nurses who worked with her, patients, family and friends who came to visit. What intrigued Saunders was that most of the traits that made Mrs. G so extraordinary emerged *after* she became ill: "Her dying had become the very means of her growth, for we learnt from her husband that her intense aliveness, gaiety and interest in other people had developed during her illness." While Saunders is clear that Mrs. G's charisma was exceptional, she also says it's not unusual for patients who are facing death to develop and grow.

"Most people who are dying still have the capacity to change in ways that are important to them," writes Ira Byock, the former hospice doctor who writes about dying. "Their transformation can also make an enormous, and lasting, difference to the people around them."

We befriended this man, Marko, who came over to the States from Croatia. You can't describe Marko: He was a very meticulous neatnik who had to be perfectly groomed at all times. He was a very old-European-manners gentleman, just a very sweet man from a whole different culture—very respectful of women. He had a terrible upbringing: He lost his only brother to suicide, he was in the war himself, and he was in illegal dealings that I never found out about, really, but toward the end, he would share about his guilt feelings.

He was a clock maker and a watch repair guy, and he got a job in New York, and then found out that he had glioblastoma, brain cancer. And they operated there. He had no money; he was some kind of public aid or charity case. Then, for some unknown reason, he answered an ad for a job in a northwest suburb of Chicago, and without telling them that he was newly post-op from brain surgery and had a basically incurable cancer, he took the new job.

It was at a jewelry store, and he lived in the apartment building right above the jeweler. Within about six months, they noticed his eyesight was going, and his balance was off. So a woman who worked with him— she was a part-time saleswoman, in her seventies— befriended Marko. She realized Marko had absolutely no one here—although he did have health insurance through the jewelry place—and she reached out to another co-worker and they both started helping out. The other woman belonged to the parish where I was parish nurse, and she came to our health committee and introduced the idea of the parish helping Marko. The parish decided to basically adopt him. We had a team of about ten people, men and women, that helped out and it became an adventure that went on for approximately three years.

During the adventure, we would have meetings, with and without Marko, the group of us, about who was doing what, who was driving him to what appointments, who was bringing food, who was doing whatever. It was really a neat thing. Marko was also a nut about cars, and the group planned a special outing for him at the Chicago auto show, which was a big deal. It's a black-tie affair with wonderful hors d'oeuvres and drinks. We got him a tux, and we dressed him up in it and we got tickets to the VIP opening, where he had the time of his life. That was a really spectacular evening.

I'm not saying it was all perfect: There were times where he got extremely difficult. At the end, he became quite paranoid. One of the younger gentlemen in our group, he was a dad in his thirties, and he was an FBI agent. Well, Marko got so paranoid, and because of things that went on in Croatia, he thought that the FBI agent was somehow spying and part of this ring trying to find him. So we went through a lot. Marko also went through a really tough time spiritually. He wasn't baptized a Catholic, but he kind of—you know, I'm not big on all the rules in the Catholic Church, and we belong to a progressive parish—and Marko just kind of pretended he was Catholic, and we all went along with it; our priest did, too.

The worst part for me of this whole story is that I had planned this Guatemala trip and it was solely a medical mission; we went there to do surgery, and it was a really neat thing that I was involved in, and we went every February. Sure enough, wouldn't you know it? He died when I was in Guatemala. I was just . . . I'll never forget that. We didn't have any cell phones at that time—there was nothing like that. So I was outside by this children's rec park in Guatemala and there was one pay phone that someone showed me how to work, and I called and found out he'd died. I felt left out; it wasn't—Marko was very well taken care of, and hospice was there, some of the group were there, so he really had a peaceful death at the end. I remember hanging up that phone and looking up—it was at night, the sky was black, black, and the moon and the stars, and I just felt really connected to him at that moment. I remember going off to a field at this place and staring up at the sky

*and thinking, "Good job, to everybody—and what a gift
Marko was to people."*—DEB CALLAHAN, HOSPICE NURSE
AND VOLUNTEER

POSTTRAUMATIC GROWTH

The "idea that great good can come from great suffering is ancient," psychologists Richard Tedeschi and Lawrence Calhoun write. Themes about the growth that can stem from suffering thread their way through Christianity, Buddhism, Islam, and Hinduism. What's relatively new is the systematic research in psychology that supports this idea. In 1996, Tedeschi and Calhoun coined the term *posttraumatic growth*, which they define as "the experience of positive change that occurs as a result of the struggle with highly challenging life crises."

A significant percentage of people who experience trauma report at least some positive outcomes from dealing with it. Depending on the criteria, Tedeschi and Calhoun estimate that between 30 and 90 percent of people who have encountered traumas say they experience some growth. "The evidence is overwhelming that individuals facing a wide variety of very difficult circumstances experience significant changes in their lives that they view as highly positive," they write.

The researchers define *trauma* or *life crisis* as circumstances that significantly challenge people's abilities to adapt, and shake up their understanding of the world and their own roles—"truly traumatic circumstances rather than everyday stressors." Researchers have seen positive changes in people who have experienced a wide spectrum of life crises: refugees and hostages; soldiers after combat; victims of sexual assault or abuse; parents who have lost a child or people whose wives, husbands, or partners have died; and patients diagnosed with serious and life-threatening diseases. But while there are several studies of posttraumatic growth in connection with serious diseases, there's much less research that deals specifically with growth and dying. Therefore, the studies cited below are based mainly on groups of trauma survivors, although palliative care professionals also report stories about the growth and development they see in individual dying patients.

First, another caveat.

DON'T *EXPECT* GROWTH FROM A CRISIS

Just as researchers warn not to expect patients to *cope* in superhuman ways, they also caution that you shouldn't expect yourself or other people to *grow* after a trauma. It would be a horrible distortion of the whole idea of posttraumatic growth if trauma survivors felt they had somehow failed because they didn't achieve it, Tedeschi and Calhoun write. The possibility of a silver lining does not make a trauma less awful, and people shouldn't view disturbing events as simply chances to grow. They refer to Rabbi Harold Kushner, who wrote about losing his son, Aaron:

> I am a more sensitive person, a more effective pastor, a more sympathetic counselor because of Aaron's life and death than I would ever have been without it. And I would give up all of those gains in a second if I could have my son back. If I could choose, I would forgo all of the spiritual growth and depth which has come my way because of our experiences, and be what I was fifteen years ago, an average rabbi, an indifferent counselor, helping some people and unable to help others, and the father of a bright, happy boy. But I cannot choose.

Even when people grow and develop after a trauma, their suffering may not diminish. In fact, people sometimes exhibit posttraumatic growth and posttraumatic stress disorder at the same time. Not everyone finds this kind of personal growth, or necessarily should find it. In the cases of some trauma sufferers, research says personal development may not be possible. And even for those who do grow, it usually takes time.

HOW POSTTRAUMATIC GROWTH WORKS

Tedeschi and Calhoun outline the process of posttraumatic growth this way: Everyone has a set of beliefs about the way the world works, their places in it, and their identities. Those beliefs guide everyday decisions and actions and allow people to function. But if catastrophe strikes, it may shatter those beliefs. In the wake of the catastrophe, some people can rebuild a set of beliefs that makes them more resilient, that allows them to connect and empathize more deeply with others, and that generally serves them better.

Growth doesn't usually start right away, the researchers write. Immediately after a trauma, most people live through a difficult period in which they just try to manage. They spend time processing what has happened to them. Then, as distress gradually ebbs, some are able to change in positive ways.

Psychologists are in rough agreement about the kinds of changes involved. Tedeschi and Calhoun categorize them into five main areas:

- People find a greater sense of strength, often because they feel that if they can rise to meet the challenge of this trauma, then surely they can face other, smaller challenges.
- People discover a new appreciation of life, and a change in priorities.

- They create warmer, more intimate relationships with others, which may include greater empathy for other suffering people, especially those who have experienced similar traumas.
- People recognize new possibilities in their lives. They may decide to pursue a different career path or hobby.
- Finally, they often come to a deeper spirituality, and even those who aren't religious may find themselves engaging more with existential questions.

Trauma survivors who experience this positive change will say things like, "I am much stronger than I ever imagined," Tedeschi and Calhoun write, or, "If I am living through this, I can live through just about anything." The researchers describe a senior executive who said his serious cancer and difficult treatments had led him to move beyond superficial pleasantries with his colleagues at work. He started talking with them about his cancer treatments and how those affected him. His colleagues, in turn, began talking with him about more profound subjects, and they were able to tell him how much they cared about his suffering. Ultimately, breaking through to these deeper, more personal conversations led to close friendships between the man and some of his colleagues.

Another man Tedeschi and Calhoun describe changed his life significantly after experiencing a serious heart attack, letting go of some of his corporate goals and prioritizing time at home with his two young children. Another patient, whose son had committed suicide, told the researchers, "I am permanently wounded, a man who will never be whole again. But I am also stronger than I thought I would be, and I find my heart going out to parents whose children suffer or other parents who have had to face the kind of hell I have been forced to live in. Maybe I can use my pain to somehow help others live through theirs."

A catastrophe doesn't lead everyone to become wiser, deeper, or more compassionate. So what makes it more likely that a particular person will grow? Researchers have found that extroverts and people who are open to experience tend to be more likely to experience posttraumatic growth. Also, optimists, although only slightly. People with strong social support. Younger people, typically, although people of all ages have developed after traumas. No matter who they are, people don't usually set out to grow from traumas. They're just trying to get through their hardships, to survive their struggles.

POSTTRAUMATIC GROWTH AND LIFE-THREATENING DISEASES

One factor in whether people experience posttraumatic growth is how significant the trauma they suffer is. A crisis needs to be serious enough to pose a threat to personal identity and deeply held beliefs. In fact, up to a certain point, the worse the perceived catastrophe, the more a person has the chance to develop.

While in one study, patients with fatal diseases or stage 4 cancer experienced less growth than people who had been through other kinds of traumas, perhaps because the trauma was so overwhelming that they mentally shut down, or perhaps because they had less time for mental processing, multiple studies show that most people diagnosed with advanced or life-threatening diseases do seem to grow and develop at least somewhat. For instance, when researchers have studied the survivors of breast cancer, testicular cancer, and bone marrow transplants, they've found that the majority experience posttraumatic growth. A study of patients who had undergone cancer surgery found that many said they had more rewarding relationships, a greater appreciation for life, and clearer priorities.

In a 2000 study of twenty-four women with breast cancer, several patients said the disease was the best thing that had ever happened to them. Many saw the cancer as a wake-up call that reminded them of what was most important in life. One said cancer had served as a door to inner wisdom; another said, "It has really given me a better knowledge of what it means to live one day at a time, what it means to appreciate what you have right now."

A 2007 study found that some participants with life-threatening illnesses came to an increased sense of well-being. For instance, one patient with multiple serious medical conditions tells researchers: "If you look from the outside, [my illness] is a bad experience. But it brought me to another point of view about life, about what's really important and what is not." Through her suffering, she says, she came to a more fulfilling sense of spirituality, understanding better what life meant to her: "Why are we here? We are here for a certain period of time. We have some things to do and in my case I think it's to take care of my children and bring them to adulthood in the safest way." This patient voices a recurring theme in the study: The very trauma that patients endured sometimes led them to find deeper meaning and to experience connectedness.

"I wouldn't be who I am today and [I wouldn't] *like* who I am today, if I had not had cancer," a forty-six-year-old woman with both colon and lung cancer, tells the researchers. "Look at how much I have learned, and grown and changed . . . it was a chance to evolve spiritually."

Gary Rodin, the psychiatrist who works with advanced cancer patients, says he and his colleagues have seen people address and even solve long-standing problems. Byock says he has observed "quantum leaps in personal development" in dying patients. Dying people sometimes find a new urgency to face old issues. Time is limited, and patients' problems become more critical. "You may have had a relationship which was workable enough, but now becomes not workable enough when your needs are very different," Rodin explains. In response, some patients and their partners will work on old issues, uncovering new depths and intimacy in their relationships. The idea that people might continue to evolve as they die is critical, some palliative care experts say. Maybe if we thought of dying as the last *stage* of life rather than merely an ending, we'd be more likely to see it as organic to human development. Maybe that would help us change the way we think about life after a fatal diagnosis.

DYING AS A LIFE STAGE

Psychologist Erik Erikson divided human lives into eight developmental stages, based roughly on age categories. According to this theory, people face a crisis and an important developmental task in each phase. If all goes well, you complete the task in one phase and then take a step forward into the next stage of development. For instance, between the time you're born and when you're one year old, the crisis you face is trust. If you have parents or caregivers who provide a sense of stability and are able to consistently make you feel safe, you usually develop a sense of trust in future relationships.

In the second stage, between the ages of roughly eighteen months and three years, you face a crisis of autonomy. Your task is to achieve some control over yourself and your environment in areas like learning how to use the toilet, learning how to choose your own food, clothes, and toys. In stage three, your crisis is between initiative and guilt. In the fourth stage, you face a crisis of industry. In this stage, your task is to learn a sense of confident competence.

The fifth stage is adolescence, and your task is finding your identity: "I have a teenager so I can see him going through this," says Virginia Lee, the nurse researcher who works with advanced cancer patients. "He thinks that he has a lot more freedom and he's trying to search for his identity with his friends and trying to move out but then there's still this sense of vulnerability where he has to stay close to the family."

In your sixth stage, you face a crisis of intimacy, and your task is to find love with a compatible partner. In the seventh stage of mature adulthood, when you're in your forties, fifties, and sixties, you face a crisis of stagnation. Your task in this stage is what Erikson calls generativity—creating something to outlast your own life, such as working to change your community, or mentoring younger people. Finally, during what's traditionally the last developmental stage, you reflect on your past. Your task is finding satisfaction with the life you've lived, and through that contentment, wisdom.

No matter what your age when you learn you have a fatal condition, the chapter of life that starts then is its own developmental period. Palliative care specialists have built on this developmental understanding to help people facing their own deaths see dying as a part of a natural progression, the last part of human development.

Just as in other life stages, dying people can grow and develop. They also face challenges. Growing in response to personal crises is hard at each stage, but perhaps most difficult in the dying stage. Continuing to develop at this stage of life almost certainly means enduring some suffering.

Thinking of dying as a life stage "doesn't mean we have to love it," says palliative care specialist James Hallenbeck. "I'm pretty sure it's not going to be the most fun stage of my life." But life stages don't exist in isolation, Hallenbeck points out. They exist in relation to other life stages. And since each stage comes with associated tasks, he asks, "If dying is, for many people, not an event anymore but a life stage—what comes with that?"

Building on Erikson's stages, Byock has created a list of

ten developmental landmarks for dying people, each with associated tasks. The landmarks include a sense of completion with worldly affairs and relationships in the community and with others; love of self and love of others; acceptance of life's finality; a sense of a new self, a sense of meaning about life in general, and a surrender to the transcendent, a letting-go.

BYOCK'S LIST OF TEN LANDMARKS AND TASKS FOR DYING PEOPLE

---

1. A sense of completion about material subjects: This includes getting finances and wills and official responsibilities in order.
2. A sense of completion about community social relationships. This includes saying formal good-byes, asking forgiveness, and expressing gratitude with people such as fellow employees, acquaintances, or others in a religious community.
3. A sense of meaning about your life. This means examining your life's major events and accomplishments and passing important stories and advice along.
4. Recognizing your love for yourself. This includes forgiving yourself for past misdeeds or failures, and acknowledging yourself.
5. Recognizing your love for others.
6. A sense of completion in close relationships.
7. A sense of acceptance of your own mortality.
8. A sense of your new identity, as a person who is still important despite a terminal diagnosis.
9. A sense of meaning about life. This includes finding a "sense of awe," of recognition that something exists beyond this life.
10. A sense of surrender to something or someone greater than yourself.

Still, dying is very individual, Byock emphasizes. The landmarks don't happen in a particular order, and not everyone experiences them all. Byock has observed people from many different backgrounds as they've faced these landmark tasks. "Each individual is on a different point in the trajectory of their illness," he writes. "Each person represents distinct demographics, culture, personal styles, tastes, and politics." Yet they share a very similar set of tasks they want to accomplish at the end of life: They all have things they want to say to the people closest to them. They each want to make out a will. They want to tell stories from their lives, to be sure those memories are preserved for family members. And even though many of his patients don't attend church, they all describe themselves as spiritual in some way.

How is it that some dying patients find this kind of healing and growth, while others don't? When people are faced with a fatal diagnosis and the prospect of dying, Hallenbeck says many are much quicker to focus on seeking a miracle cure than to ask, "How do I do this?" If more of us could see dying as something we *do,* rather than something that is *done to* us, we'd be more likely to experience development, he says.

DIGNITY FOR DYING PEOPLE

Early in his career, psychiatrist Harvey Chochinov and his colleagues at the University of Manitoba noticed how often people talked about the importance of dying with dignity. The most common reason cited for patients wishing to hasten their own deaths was loss of dignity. But he found no studies defining what, exactly, people meant by the term as it applied to dying people.

"If dignity was worth dying for, then dignity was worth studying," he concluded. So Chochinov and his colleagues asked fifty patients who had been diagnosed with fatal diseases what they thought: How do you define dignity? What supports your sense of dignity, and what takes away from it?

The patients talked about the ways their illnesses threatened their dignity, but they also talked about how they were sometimes able to conserve dignity through their own attitudes or actions. The patients kept returning to the idea of generativity, the task of stage seven/late adulthood according to Erikson's eight developmental stages and tasks. Patients wanted to generate—to create—some kind of legacy. How they were remembered was especially important to them: "Will my life, and the meaning of my life, continue to resonate in the minds of the people that I leave behind?" they would ask. "What will my life have stood for? What is the meaning of my existence? Will there be ripple effects after I'm gone?"

Chochinov and his colleagues set about trying to find a method to help dying people create a legacy. What they came up with was a method they called "dignity therapy." The protocol starts with an introductory session, which is followed by a recorded session. In this second session, the therapist begins by asking the patient: "Tell me a little about your life history, particularly the parts that you either remember most or think are the most important? When did you feel most alive?"

The therapist follows that initial question with others like, "Are there specific things that you would want your family to know about you, and are there particular things you would want them to remember?" and "What have you learned about life that you would want to pass along to others? What advice or words of guidance would you wish to pass along?"

The guided reflections work well because dying patients tend to have a kind of "existential readiness," Chochinov says: "There are times in our lives, whether we're imminently dying, or particularly ill, or we're faced with the possibility of a life-threatening condition, when reflection and looking back becomes important." Chochinov's therapy provides suggested questions, but these are just a framework. The sessions vary according to the patients. "For some it may be very much about storytelling, and about talking about their families and talking about important reminiscences," Chochinov says. Others seek forgiveness or want to express feelings they hope others will take away from their life experiences. In some cases, people have used the sessions to give their spouses permission to remarry or find happiness with another partner.

The recording is then transcribed, and here's the part I like the best: It's edited. First, interruptions are removed and any needed clarifications are made. Next, the transcription is edited for chronology. If events in a patient's life are recounted out of order but would make better sense told chronologically, those changes are made.

Then, any content that might cause significant emotional harm for family members is omitted or tagged, and these sections are discussed with the patient. "Words are powerful," Chochinov says, underscoring that he wants to be sure that whatever is created is respectful of family members' feelings. "The only way to do that was by being sure that there was an opportunity to help guide patients through content that might potentially be difficult for family members to hear, or to know about."

The editor tries to be sure the transcript ends with a statement that fits with the patient's overall message.

The document is then read to the patient, and most of the time, further changes are minimal. "Occasionally, depending on the patient and the circumstances, they might say, 'There's something more that I need included,' and there may be another session set up," Chochinov says.

The final edited document is given to patients to do with as they see fit—usually to give to family members as a legacy. The goal is to provide the version that patients want their family members to have as a remembrance, Chochinov says.

"I suppose at the end of life, we all have ways of looking back and editing and revising, and revisiting different chapters and looking at them perhaps in different ways." Dignity therapy provides a material way for patients to pass that along to their families. Sometimes, the narratives might not seem especially profound to outsiders, but the dying people and their families know that the memories and advice are uniquely personal. Chochinov describes one patient who "was just overwhelmed when he looked at the document and realized that it kind of captured the essence of who he was and the things that he wanted said to his wife and family, and the advice that he gave."

For another patient, the crucial point was communicating a message. He had two children in his first marriage, but he later divorced and remarried. "One of the important tasks that he felt dignity therapy needed to serve was to try and provide, not so much an apology—but some kind of an explanation to his children as to why he had left this relationship," Chochinov says. He wanted them "to know that leaving the marriage wasn't leaving behind the care and the love that he felt towards these children."

For another patient, a woman with metastatic breast cancer, dignity therapy helped her create a document that she'd been trying unsuccessfully to write on her own. Chochinov remembers the woman telling him that she had tried over and over to write down the story of her life for her children and grandchildren but found the task overwhelming. She didn't know where to begin her story, or how to organize it, although she felt it was crucial to communicate her sense of how close the family had been so they could continue that tradition after she had died.

People might intuitively expect that the therapy is for those who have had especially adventuresome, successful, or interesting lives and therefore have incredible stories to tell, but

Chochinov has found that everyone has a story. Some of them may be grand, some may be tragic, or maybe even funny. But the only person who can tell the story is that individual, because they are unique, and they've lived it.

A FATAL DIAGNOSIS DOESN'T MEAN LIFE IS FINISHED

When the famous neurologist Oliver Sacks learned he had terminal cancer, he wrote in a *New York Times* opinion piece that he didn't see his life as finished: "On the contrary, I feel intensely alive, and I want and hope in the time that remains to deepen my friendships, to say farewell to those I love, to write more, to travel if I have the strength, to achieve new levels of understanding and insight."

For people with a terminal disease, time becomes suspended in slow motion, allowing them the chance to grow and develop at a faster rate than at any other time in their lives. Saunders says: "We see people go through a lifetime of experience in a few weeks, a long time is fulfilled in a short time. They seem to know a timeless 'Now' when all the moments of time are held in stillness."

People shouldn't expect victims of trauma to grow or be heroic, but when a person is facing death, she needs to know that possibility exists. And the people around her need to allow for it.

Like other dying patients, and like the people who care for them, Sacks, who was eighty-one when he received his terminal diagnosis, knew he was tackling a big challenge: "This will involve audacity, clarity and plain speaking; trying to straighten my accounts with the world," he writes.

"But there will be time, too, for some fun (and even some silliness, as well)."

chapter eight

checking out early

MY FAMILY ASSUMED we'd have months between my mother's decision to suspend her chemo treatments and her death. A procession of out-of-town friends and relatives would visit. We'd travel to somewhere exotic, or at least spend a weekend in nearby Santa Fe or Telluride. We'd share one last spring together.

What we had instead was three weeks.

Despite the unexpected beauty and sanctity of that time, we wished it were half as long. My mother was ready to die. Later, after her death, we would agonize with each other about her last episode of severe pain. My brother said we should have found a way to help her end her life sooner, and we wondered aloud about researching the subject before our own deaths.

My mother's life was infinitely precious to us. In those brief conversations when we broached the topic of hastening her death—there were two, I think, both after she died—we had no idea where we would have started. If we'd asked, would anyone have told us which drugs we needed to end her suffering, and where or how we could have obtained them?

ASKING A NURSE OR DOCTOR TO HELP
HASTEN DEATH

"I've had a number of patients on the hospice program who say, 'Look, Doc, I've had it. I have pancreatic cancer. I don't want to put my family through this anymore,'" says Fred Schwartz, the medical director of Hospice New York. "'Give me the shot of morphine and let me go. I'm ready, I'm set, my family is going to support me.'"

Schwartz, who also sits on the board of End of Life Choices New York, has to tell them, "I hear you, but I can't do that."

Judith Schwarz, the clinical director at End of Life Choices New York—she is unrelated to Fred Schwartz and spells her last name differently—has had similar experiences: "Everybody wants the magic purple pill: 'I'm available this afternoon—could you bring it this afternoon so I can just go to sleep and not wake up?'

"And I say, 'I understand that that's what you would like to do.'" But medical aid in dying is still illegal in most states, including New York. Furthermore, there's no such pill.

But that doesn't keep some family members or patients from asking medical professionals to help them with an early exit.

Even in cases where medical professionals can legally assist dying patients in hastening death—or legally provide advice and support—their first response is to look for and treat underlying problems. Schwarz describes a conversation with a recent patient who had stage 4 lung cancer: "She said, 'I want to die because I can't stand the nausea I'm experiencing.'" The woman had a symptom that was understandably difficult—even intolerable—but it was treatable, so Schwarz told her, "We need to get your nausea controlled; we need to get better palliative care . . . Because, if you're in terrible pain, or if you're terribly nauseated, of course you want to die. So let's see if we can get those symptoms relieved, so that you can actually make a thoughtful choice."

Once terminally ill patients receive significant pain relief or psychological support, their desire to end their lives early often disappears. But not always.

"IT'S NOT ABOUT PAIN"

Schwarz remembers when a close friend called her after years of enduring multiple rounds of chemotherapy and radiation for her ovarian cancer. The friend was in pain, and asked Schwarz to help her die. "She said, 'I can't do this anymore. You've got to help me: I want to know how I can die. This is too much. I can't deal with this pain.' And so I just rode right over, and I thought, 'Oh, I can take care of that. We'll just get her pain under control, and then she won't want to die.' And that was my first introduction to *you think it's simple?* It's not simple."

Schwarz would come to realize that her friend's deteriorating quality of life caused her even greater suffering than her physical pain. The friend would later agree to one more surgery, hoping to enjoy a last holiday with her family. But the outcome of the surgery was not what she had hoped for, and she returned home on hospice care. "She said, 'Okay, fine, that's it,'" Schwarz says. She was ready to die.

Over time, Schwarz has learned that pain is not the main reason most patients want to end their lives early. "It's not about pain," she says. "It would be nice if you're *not* in pain, but that's not why people want to die."

Patients typically have multiple reasons for seeking a hastened death, including pain, other physical symptoms, loss of meaning, and fear of becoming a burden. People who intentionally hasten their deaths "are doing so because they find some aspect of the process of dying intolerable," Schwarz says. "They're suffering because of the manner in which they're dying."

While hastening dying is still controversial in most places, the artificial lengthening of lives through technology and modern medicine has brought a greater tolerance for it. Dying patients who end their lives early are all seeking something similar, Schwarz says: "What people want at the end of life is to not get stuck, to not get trapped in an endlessly intolerable dying experience—that's what people are afraid of.

"They're afraid of the dehumanizing aspects of dying on a machine or being trapped in a body that they can't control, or losing their mind, or all of these things. And so, what they want to know is that they have options, that they have choices."

"YOU'VE GOT PLENTY OF STUFF IN THE HOUSE"

Schwarz's friend would later ask her again to help end her life early. That experience of being asked to help someone end her life early led Schwarz to wonder about other nurses. Surely they, too, had received similar requests.

Ten nurses eventually agreed to fill out Schwarz's anonymous survey by describing their experiences. They'd all had at least one patient ask for help in hastening death: "Usually the way the question was framed, in this very sort of careful voice by family members, was, 'What would happen if I gave a little bit more, a little bit more often?'" Schwarz says. She found that nurses' responses to these requests fell into a classic bell-shaped curve:

On one end, were the ones that said, "Are you out of your mind? Absolutely not. I wouldn't help you with that. That's illegal" . . . And, on the other extreme, were those who said, "I'll write you a prescription. We'll figure out how to do this . . . This is your right. I'll help you with it." And most of them were muddling around in the middle: "I'm not sure. Um, er, Is this right? Is this wrong? Can I do this? Can I not? Am I helping? Am I not helping?"

Nurses, who are the most likely to be the hands-on medical professionals attending to dying patients, are often caught in the middle, between a wish to ease patients' suffering, and their professional and ethical values. Several told Schwarz they gave some version of the following response to patient or family requests for aid in dying: "You can do whatever you think is right. It's up to you. You've got plenty of stuff in the house."

What they meant, she says, is that hospice typically stocks the homes of dying patients with strong painkillers such as liquid morphine, oxycodone, methadone, or fentanyl. The drugs are there in case a patient's pain suddenly spikes.

Nobody seems to know how commonly this happens, but every now and then, patients and family members decide to use the medication in understandable but illegal ways, says Peter Rogatz, the former director of the Long Island Jewish Medical Center and a cofounder of End of Life Choices New York. "Patients get morphine in solution from a hospice program quite typically, with the instruction to the caregiver, who is probably a spouse or a son or a daughter, to give [the patient] a teaspoon of this once every three hours or so. If he's in pain, if he's in a lot of pain, you could give him a little more," Rogatz says. "Well, you don't have to say more than that to a family member who is distressed about the patient being distressed."

It's important to remember that morphine, or other opiates, aren't particularly dangerous medicines when administered in a medical setting, especially for dying patients, Rogatz emphasizes. "Morphine is a very, very appropriate drug to be getting toward the end of life," he says, and medical professionals can be pretty certain how much of an opiate is safe.

But even if they wanted to do the opposite of what they're trained to do—if their goal was to kill the dying patient—

medical professionals would usually have difficulty calculating how much to administer. Schwarz says: "Most people don't know what a lethal dose is, because that's not something you teach in either nursing or medical school."

The number of tragic overdoses among drug addicts often makes people wonder why using opioids to hasten dying would be difficult, says Terry Law, a medical adviser for End of Life Washington. "You think, why is it so hard to kill these people when these drug addicts do it all the time, right? But they're injecting. It's almost impossible to get a fatal dose of morphine orally," she says. The drug has to be absorbed through the stomach and metabolized by the liver, both of which are usually functioning poorly in dying patients.

Furthermore, as an opioid is administered, a patient's tolerance grows, so the amount needed to dull pain or other symptoms also increases. "Anybody who has been on opiates for any length of time develops a tolerance to the central nervous system's side effects," Schwarz says, "so it is damn-near impossible to kill yourself with opiates if you've been on opiates for any length of time, unless you have a huge amount that you can inject [through an] IV."

Still, there are stories of dying patients who manage to use the drugs at home to end their lives early. Nurses who tell family members there are plenty of potent drugs in the house are indicating, both through what they say and what they don't say, that they would look the other way if someone purposely gave the patient a lethal dose of drugs. But is this the right thing to do? "What they're doing is morally abandoning these family members," Schwarz says. "This is really hard stuff for a family member to do."

Schwarz believes medical professionals should never abandon their patients. Instead, they should work to provide better symptom management. They should listen and try to understand how best to help. If they live in a place where aid in dying is legal, they can explain to patients how the law works, she says. And no matter where someone lives, there are legal ways for patients to hasten their own deaths.

VOLUNTARILY STOPPING EATING AND DRINKING

In his role as a hospice medical director, Fred Schwartz says that every now and then—perhaps twice a year—he works with a dying patient who is determined to end life early. If that patient's pain and symptoms are under control with the best means available, and if it's clear the patient is decision-ally capable—that is, over the age of eighteen, mentally sound, and able to make good decisions—and is not depressed, then Schwartz may tell the patient: "One of the things you can do, and this is perfectly your choice, is to stop eating and drinking."

Advocates point out that voluntarily stopping eating and drinking, or VSED, is legal across the United States and in most Western countries, and it gives the patient some control over dying—as opposed to needing a prescription from a doctor and having to meet the strict requirements in states that allow medically assisted dying.

But no one takes the idea lightly. VSED, while not painful, is also not easy.

"The business of dying is not easy, and I don't think it should be easy, actually," Judith Schwarz says. Deciding to hasten your death "needs to be a thoughtful, clearly, well-considered decision. I do not support suicide, and I really make a big distinction between suicide and somebody who's hastening an inevitable death because their current situation is intolerable."

Sometimes, patients want to give up eating and drinking without telling anyone else, she says. "They're just going to take care of this themselves—just tell them how they can do it. And I say, 'You can't do it by yourself. You absolutely cannot do this by yourself.'"

The beginning of the VSED process is especially challenging and requires a lot of support, explains Rogatz. The first few days are usually uncomfortable. "It's not excruciating, but there are hunger pangs and there's thirst, thirst being the more difficult of the two," he says. "A patient who is in hospice will be sedated sufficiently, just enough to take the edge off of the thirst and the hunger. [In fact,] I don't know of any patient who's accomplished this without being in hospice."

Schwarz says VSED patients who are enrolled in hospice are far more likely to meet the goal of hastening their own deaths. She gives a long list of reasons as to why that's true:

> You end up being in bed around the clock. You can't get up by yourself to go to the bathroom or you'll fall down and break a hip. You're going to be in diapers. You're going to have to have 24/7 caregiving help at some point. You need psychosocial support—people who understand why you've made this choice, and we'll kind of help you over the rough spots. Going without food is pretty easy; going without fluids can be a real challenge. It can be really, really hard. And you have to have people who are knowledgeable about giving really good oral care and helping you rinse and spit, reminding you not to swallow, and trying different things to keep you comfortable. You have to have access to good palliative medical oversight. You have to have access to small doses of morphine, small doses of liquid morphine, liquid Ativan, anti-anxiety medication.

The patients who successfully use VSED to hasten death are determined and well informed, Schwarz says. Ideally, they've laid the groundwork months or years ahead of time in checkups with their regular physician. They've talked with family members so everyone knows and supports the plan.

They've made sure they have access to good medical care, and to home health aides who will support VSED. Then, if and when the time comes, they're more likely to be ready to give up eating and drinking.

HOW VSED WORKS

"What's it like? It depends," says Schwarz. In the first few days, which are the hardest, "the goal is to have you in kind of a sleepy, sort of semi-wakeful state." That helps dull pangs of hunger and thirst. VSED is different from naturally losing your appetite and thirst, which happens to many dying patients as a physiological response to active dying.

In contrast, when patients voluntarily stop eating and drinking, their bodies usually take longer to adapt. As a general rule, hunger doesn't cause much hardship in this scenario, and the sensation disappears after about twenty-four hours. Thirst is much more difficult, although it's still treatable. Patients' mouths can be rinsed with water or a moist swab; their lips can be moistened with lip balm. If they decide to do any more than that—if patients drink even a little water—dying takes longer, Rogatz says. "Stopping eating and drinking has to be taken very literally. You can't say, 'Well, I'll just take a sip of water every once in a while.' That slows the process considerably," he explains. "I would say if the patient is taking more than a half a teaspoon of liquid during the course of a day, they are slowing the process."

For a person who gives up eating and drinking, active dying starts when the kidneys shut down. And in order to shut down, the kidneys must stop receiving fluids, Rogatz says. "It's interesting: The kidneys don't need a lot of liquid to function, and they really have to be pretty well deprived," he explains. "What happens is, the volume of blood in the body is reduced and that's what produces the physiologic signal to the kidneys to start shutting down."

Some VSED patients change their minds, and if they do, caregivers have to respect that choice, Schwarz says— although caregivers sometimes remind patients about their earlier decisions if the patients' memories have become muddled. Sometimes, what patients crave is just the idea of food and liquid. Schwarz worked with one woman who had given up eating and drinking but then developed a sudden thirst for a favorite drink.

One day, I get a panic call from one of the daughters, who says, "Oh my god, Mom just woke up and said she wants a margarita. What should we do?"

I said, "Give her a margarita."

She said, "Really?"

I said, "Yeah. Make it exactly as she wants, and hold it out for her, and I bet she'll have a sip, and she'll close her eyes and then go back to sleep."

And that's exactly what happened.

After a few days without food or liquid, most patients start to fall into a coma, although the length of time depends on the patient's original condition. "It's gradual; it starts around the third, fourth, fifth day," Rogatz says. Most patients completely lose consciousness by the sixth or eighth day. After that, as far as anyone can tell, they don't feel anything.

The time between when a person first gives up food and liquids, and death, is longer than most people initially think: Ten to fourteen days is typical, although the interval can range from six to twenty-four days.

The process can be longer for athletes because they have strong cardiovascular systems; it tends to be shorter for patients who are already weak and have lost a lot of weight.

Schwarz says it's easiest to predict how long the process will take for cancer patients. "I can usually tell, once I see someone," she says. For most cancer patients, it's about ten days. While this method of hastening death is significantly longer than others, the vast majority of reported deaths through VSED are peaceful, with little suffering. Still, Schwarz has seen some patients struggle. Sometimes, they don't really understand how serious the process is or aren't sufficiently determined. In some cases, patients experience terminal agitation: "As the organs begin to fail and no longer function effectively, they can no longer detoxify what's in your body and things like morphine don't get broken down and excreted as well, and there can be some buildup in that," she explains. "And one of the side effects of that is agitation and delirium, which is a terrible experience to witness." Haldol has proven a very effective drug for treating this kind of agitation and delirium, Schwarz says.

In other cases, dealing with thirst or hunger is torturous for patients. "It's one of the questions I always ask people, 'Do you still have an appetite? Are you still hungry? Do you get pleasure out of eating?'" Because if the answer to any of those is *yes,* she tells them, then perhaps VSED is not the right approach.

"This is not for everyone," Schwarz emphasizes. "You know, this is not a choice for everyone."

DYING WITH MEDICAL AID

Aid in dying, in some form, is legal in Canada, the Netherlands, Belgium, Colombia, Germany, Switzerland, and Luxembourg. And in seven states in the United States, doctors can legally prescribe lethal doses of medicine to terminally ill patients. These are, in order of legalization: Oregon, Washington, Montana, Vermont, California, Colorado, and Hawaii, as well as the District of Columbia. No "death with dignity" law has been passed in Montana; medical aid in dying is legal there because of a court ruling.

Oregon, whose law was passed in 1997, has by far the most experience with how medically assisted dying works, and its health department publishes an annual report. Since the law first took effect there, 1,967 patients have received lethal prescriptions, and 1,275 have taken the medication and died as a result, according to the state's report for 2017.

The three most frequent reasons Oregon patients give for choosing medically assisted dying have remained relatively consistent over two decades: They are concerned about loss of autonomy, loss of dignity, and a lowered ability to participate fully in the activities that matter to them. Patients also say they are concerned about loss of control over bodily functions, being a burden, inadequate pain control, and, to a much lesser extent, the financial implications of treatment.

Slightly more men than women take advantage of Oregon's law. Most have at least some college education. Most are white, and most are sixty-five or older. Most, although not all, tell their families. Ninety percent have been enrolled in hospice. The disease patients are most likely to have is cancer, by a significant margin.

The requirements for medical aid in dying are similar in all seven states and the District: Patients must be residents, over eighteen, and have a terminal condition that makes it likely they will die within six months. Unlike doctors in the Netherlands, Canada, Luxembourg, Colombia, and Belgium, physicians in the United States are not allowed to administer doses with an intention to kill patients. Instead, the aid that American doctors offer patients in dying is through writing prescriptions for lethal doses of drugs that patients must be able to administer themselves.

Two physicians must agree that the patient is eligible, and

either physician can require a psychiatric evaluation if he or she believes it might be warranted. Patients must wait fifteen days after their initial request for a lethal prescription, and then make a second request. They must also make a written request. Doctors are required to fill out reports when they consult or prescribe in cases of medically assisted dying. But there is nothing in the laws on medically assisted dying about what kinds of drugs they can or should prescribe.

"THERE AREN'T ANY STUDIES ON HOW TO KILL PEOPLE"

In countries where physicians are allowed to administer lethal medications, the problem of which drug to use is simpler. When doctors inject drugs, they can use higher doses and they don't need to worry about whether patients will be able to absorb the drugs through the intestinal tract, or will vomit when they swallow them. In the Netherlands, for instance, most physicians use thiopental to place their aid-in-dying patients in a coma, and then inject a neuromuscular blocker. In Canada, physicians also usually administer a mixture of drugs to sedate patients and put them into a coma, and then inject a neuromuscular blocker.

In places like the United States, where aid-in-dying patients are required to take their medications orally themselves, the most frequently used drugs until recently were either pentobarbital or secobarbital, both originally prescribed as sleeping medications. But pentobarbital became mostly unavailable in U.S. pharmacies in 2015, perhaps because it was being used even in oral form for capital punishment and the European manufacturer objected, although no one seems certain. In the same year, the price of secobarbital jumped suddenly: When Sue Dessayer Porter, the founding executive director of End of Life Choices Oregon, first began working with terminally ill patients in 2000, secobarbital cost about $130, she says. Now, the same amount costs about $3,500.

After the price increase, an informal group of concerned doctors in Oregon and Washington began searching for a more affordable option. Terry Law, the End of Life Washington medical adviser, was one of the doctors doing the research. "There aren't any studies on how to kill people," she says. "We looked through the literature to see if we could find medications that were almost universally fatal." At first, they tried a compound with chloral hydrate that seemed to work well. But caregivers and volunteers expressed dismay at the pain and discomfort that sometimes accompanied ingesting the medication: It burned patients' throats and had a particularly vile taste. So the doctors came up with a more promising combination, DDMP: diazepam, digoxin, morphine, and propranolol. Diazepam—originally sold as Valium—is a drug used for conditions such as anxiety or insomnia. Together with morphine, high doses of the drug induce a coma. Propranolol and digoxin are cardiac drugs that, in large doses, slow or stop the heart. The group later tweaked this compound when they discovered it sometimes took longer to take effect, causing added anxiety for caregivers. Dosage recommendations were increased, and the new combination was dubbed DDMP2.

This compound and secobarbital are now the medications used for most aid in dying in the United States.

STARTING THE PROCESS

Once patients make the decision to seek medical assistance in dying, they need to be determined, says Porter: "Going through the process is obtuse; it is difficult; it is a hassle." Patients who choose medical aid in dying—or simply choose to have a prescription filled that they never use—say the legislation brings a sense of relief, a reassurance that their suffering won't be prolonged. But the laws are imperfect. Porter says the focus of her graduate thesis was on how the Oregon legislation should be changed. And Lonny Shavelson, the founder of Bay Area End of Life Options in Berkeley, California, is critical of the way other states have copied Oregon's death-with-dignity law and traditions, despite the fact that the law is over twenty years old. For instance, the medications are much less predictable and potent because the laws don't allow injections, Shavelson says. He also objects to the fact that the laws allow any doctor to write prescriptions for aid in dying; in an ideal world, this would protect vulnerable patients by ensuring that they were tended by someone who knew them well. But in practice, Shavelson says, it means doctors who have little to no experience are supposed to help patients in an area that does require expertise.

Shavelson's organization, which includes another doctor and a nurse, is rare in that it openly advises patients about end-of-life options and also prescribes the medications, if patients request them and he feels they are appropriate. He has assisted seventy-three patients with medical aid in dying, and he says these have been good deaths that have ultimately brought peace to dying patients. But because of flaws in both the legislation and practices, the process of getting there has often been a struggle.

Usually, the first difficulty patients encounter is the search for a doctor willing to participate. While surveys in Europe and the United States have been limited and imperfect, they have shown doctors trailing the rest of the population in their support for aid in dying: In the United Kingdom, France, Italy, Germany, and Spain, 47 percent or fewer of surveyed physicians supported aid in dying. The majority of U.S. doctors say they are in favor of medically assisted dying, but in practice, many are unwilling to prescribe lethal doses of drugs. And most of those who are willing to prescribe will only do so for their own patients. "Let's say [patients] start dialing different oncology offices, no one is going to answer the phone, saying, 'Oh yes, we do that—come on in,'" Porter says.

Law was close to retiring from her career as an internal medicine doctor when a volunteer asked her to write a lethal prescription for a patient who couldn't find anyone else to do it. Since then, she has written medical aid in dying prescriptions for 180 patients, none of whom she has charged for her services.

Even doctors who agree to help patients take advantage of the law often don't want to be the ones writing prescriptions. Instead, they'll agree to be a consulting doctor—the physician who offers a second opinion that the patient is eligible under the law. Sometimes, doctors agree in advance to write a lethal prescription, but when the time comes, they change their minds.

Shavelson says he's taken on several patients because a doctor who had previously agreed to be their prescribing doctor finally said, "I don't know how to do this. I'm not going to do it." When that happens, the patient has to start over from the beginning before the fifteen-day waiting period can begin.

That waiting period is closer to a month by the time most patients wade through the process, say both Shavelson and Porter. The intent is to prevent hasty decisions. "But nobody is suddenly thinking about it on the first day that they make the first request, and now they need fifteen days to figure it out," Shavelson says. "Every one of our patients has thought about it for a couple of years."

Depending on the state, laws differ about when patients have to sign a witnessed paper expressing their intent, and sometimes patients get confused about the timing. In Washington, doctors must wait another forty-eight hours after patients sign the form before they can write a prescription, Law says. "Then the doctor, in our state, has to hand-deliver or mail the prescription to the pharmacy. You cannot give them to family members to take to the pharmacy."

WHEN DO YOU TAKE THE MEDICATIONS?

Once patients know that their medication is sitting at a pharmacy, "it is such a relief," Porter says. "There's a sense of, 'Wow, I can get this any time.'"

That's been Law's experience with patients, too: "What we have found is once these patients know that everything's in order and they have the option, they have a sense of control—often at the end of life people have very little control—and they feel calmer about things," she says. "We hear that from families, we hear it from clients, and people just feel better, knowing that they have the option."

Sometimes, patients are eager to take the medication as soon as it's available, and Porter says all the patients with whom she's worked have at least intended to take it at some point: "Once that whole process is done and the prescription is at the pharmacy, I've never had anyone say, 'I've decided not to take it.'"

There are patients who wait for one more important life event—to visit with a grandson one last time, say, or see photos from a wedding they can't attend. For these, deciding when to take the medications can prove a high-stakes waiting game, because they must be mentally and physically capable of ingesting it themselves. As people decline in health and begin to approach death, some lose the capacity to swallow; others deteriorate mentally to the point that they no longer meet the laws' minimum qualifications for mental competence. Porter, who has worked with terminally ill patients as a case volunteer since 2000, has shown up three times for a medically assisted death, only to learn she cannot help because the patient has either lost mental capacity overnight or fallen into a coma.

In other cases, patients have lost—or been concerned they'll lose—the physical ability to take the drugs, Porter says. She recently worked with a patient who was hospitalized for a throat obstruction. Doctors told the patient that the obstruction would almost definitely recur, and if it did, she knew she wouldn't be able to swallow the medications. So she decided to take the lethal drugs right away, rather than risk not being able to take them at all.

In California, Shavelson has developed slightly different practices in writing prescriptions and assisting his patients: He offers to pick up the prescriptions from the pharmacy, and he has attended the deaths of all but one of his patients. He also waits to write the prescription until just a day or two before the date the patient has chosen to die. If the prescription is available any time, he says, "Sometimes you take it too early; sometimes, you take it too late; sometimes you take it because you stubbed your toe in the morning, your foot hurts, and you had an argument with your wife." Some patients will call him to say they're ready to die because they're in severe pain. He'll tell them, "What you have is a pain crisis. You don't have a need for aid in dying. You need to have your pain treated."

In one case, Shavelson arrived on the day a patient had decided to take the medications, only to find that the patient's condition had deteriorated severely: "I said, 'From yesterday, when we shipped you the medicines, you've progressed. And you know what? You're doing great. You don't need these medicines,'" Shavelson says. "And the patient said, 'I really want to take them.'"

But Shavelson was firm. "No, you're doing fine," he said. "You're going to die just fine; you're about to be unconscious; you're barely talking to me." The patient died a short time afterwards—without needing the prescription.

ONCE THE DAY ARRIVES

When Shavelson or one of his colleagues arrives on the day a patient is slated to take the medications, "it's a lighter atmosphere than you think—because they're less worried, knowing that we're coming," he says, and there's a palpable sense of relief. "The first thing I say to every patient is, 'Here's the deal: There are no rules for today; you get to make the rules—not me, not your family members,'" Shavelson says. "'This is your day.'"

Patients make very different choices about what that day is like. Some have music playing, Law says, while others prefer quiet. One woman arranged for a sort of British tea party, with cucumber sandwiches and high tea. Some deaths are attended only by one or two other people, while others are occasions for large family gatherings. Law recalls a death at which about twenty relatives and friends were present. "And everybody was kind of laughing and joking, and then somebody had the idea that they would all come in separately and say good-bye," she says. "About three-quarters of the way through, he said, 'I can't do this anymore.'" The patient didn't have the emotional or physical energy to deal with so many individual farewells, so the room was cleared of people while he took the medications.

In most cases in Oregon, the prescribing physician isn't present, although a hospice nurse often is, Porter says. In her experiences, neither physicians nor nurses mix the drugs or hand them to the patient. Instead, a family member or, more often an End of Life Choices volunteer like Porter, helps patients at this stage. "We don't want families to have to go through that one more emotional hurdle" of having to administer the medication, she says.

When Porter is the volunteer present, she asks the patient the following questions before she begins preparing the medicine:

First of all: "Would you like to change your mind? You have the right to change your mind."

Secondly: "What is this medication going to do?"

(I always make sure there's family or friends around so everyone hears this. And once in a while, a person will joke, but I say, "No, I'm serious, what is this medication going to do?" Until they say, "Die," or "death," I don't move forward.)

And then the third question is, "Whose decision is this?" And so everyone knows, it's their decision.

Then we prepare the medication.

When patients or their caregivers pick DDMP up at a pharmacy, the drug is in powdered form. Secobarbital comes in capsules, and a caregiver or a volunteer like Porter must open a hundred capsules and empty the powdered drug from each. For either drug, Porter says she then adds three to four ounces of water to dissolve it for patients.

Shavelson has his patients rehearse ahead of time with Ensure so they have plenty of practice in drinking four ounces of liquid in two minutes. "Why is it four ounces in two minutes?" he asks. "Because if you take longer than two minutes, you may fall asleep halfway through the dose."

Both secobarbital and DDMP2 are bitter. "They taste terrible," Law says. "So we have people use sorbet, kind of between drinks—we have them drink it through a straw to kind of get it past the taste buds—and use sorbet, or honey, or whatever they think—root beer—something to kind of mask the nasty taste."

Porter says she used to tell patients they could take the medications with applesauce, until a patient's spouse added a cherry-flavored laxative to the applesauce to make the concoction taste better. The laxative affected the chemistry of the lethal drug and the patient later woke up. Now she makes sure patients don't add anything to the prescription, although they can drink almost anything they want after they've consumed it.

Patients have only a little time after ingesting the drugs before they fall into a coma. "There's a little bit of conversation," Porter says, although usually not much. "Then you see them starting to just drift off. Or they'll say, 'Oh, I'm feeling dizzy.' Sometimes, there's someone lying by them, hugging them, and their eyes start drooping."

Shavelson says his patients usually become silent after they drink the medications. "There's just something about the moment. They've said what they're going to say by that time." For a few minutes, patients usually continue to sit silently, their eyes open. "And then, very, very slowly, they'll close their eyes."

Shavelson will ask them intermittently, "Are you still there?" and patients will usually say yes, or nod. Within five or ten minutes, patients stop responding to the question. Then Shavelson will gently touch their eyelids. "When people aren't deeply unconscious, they'll sort of have a twitching response," he explains. Within ten or fifteen minutes, the twitching response disappears and patients enter a deep coma.

Typically, they grab the cup and most of them drink it down relatively quickly. We have them sit up as high as we can and as long as they can if they're able to so it gets into their stomach, and then have them recline again. Sometimes we roll them on their right side, thinking that could help things empty into the stomach, but there's controversy about that. The patients have been saying their good-byes for a while, so a lot of times they don't say a lot. The people around them are trying not to cry, and sometimes we are, too. Recently there was a thirty-some-year-old mother with advanced cancer who had six- and eight-year-old kids, and she did an incredible job of preparing everyone. When the volunteer got there, there were quite a few people there saying good-bye. And all of a sudden, the volunteer said, the little six-year-old

came into the room and said, "Mom's getting ready to
take her medicine to go to heaven—come on!"—TERRY
LAW, MEDICAL ADVISER FOR END OF LIFE WASHINGTON

The medications are painless, and they induce unconsciousness quickly. According to Oregon state reports, most
patients become unconscious within five minutes after taking
the medication. They're in a coma, "just completely out of it,"
Porter says. "We don't know whether they can hear us or not.
I assume they can't; other people assume they can. And they
start the dying process."

It's hard to predict the time between coma and death, and
this is where the drugs' effects are less consistent. According
to the Oregon annual report, patients have usually taken a
total of about twenty-five minutes to die, although this interval has sometimes stretched to ten hours or, once, four days.
It has been as short as one minute.

Shavelson has learned that particular groups of patients
are at risk for lengthier deaths: Patients who are especially
thin and wasted from their disease, because their ability to
absorb medications has also been affected. Patients who have
been on high doses of painkillers. Athletes who have strong
hearts, even if they haven't run for five years. "We now take
athletic histories on every patient we see," Shavelson says.
If he suspects a patient is a high risk, he will change doses,
methods of administration, or even which drugs he prescribes.

A patient is scheduled for medical aid in dying on the
tenth of this month, I think that's right—it's a Saturday.
She's a wonderful person. She's fifty-two years old. She
has pancreatic cancer—risk factor one, because of the
positioning of the pancreatic cancer next to your gut; it
pushes on the gut, it delays gastric emptying into the
duodenum where absorption happens, or it obstructs

the duodenum partially. Risk factor two: She's worked out at the gym, full cardiovascular workouts, every day of her life, and she hikes. People who have strong hearts because of a long history of phenomenal exercise have tremendous pulmonary and cardiovascular conditioning. So she has pancreatic cancer, she's young, has a strong heart, has cardiovascular conditioning, and she scares the shit out of me because she has all these risk factors for taking a long time to die. So we have arrangements with her: We're going to use higher doses of medications. For the first time in a long time, I'm going to bring back chloral hydrate, which is a very foul-tasting but extremely effective medicine. We'll give that as a separate dose. She's got an eighteen-year-old kid and a husband—she doesn't want them hanging around for ten hours while she dies. We are adjusting our medications, as well as preparing the family for the possibility that this could go on for a while. We're going to do everything we can to make it short, and I think it will be, but we're also preparing in case it isn't. She has gastroparesis as well from her pancreatic cancer, so her stomach is essentially paralyzed; it's going to slowly move the meds into the duodenum. But there are medications you use to stimulate the stomach. So we're going to give her that beforehand; we're going to use higher doses of medications; we're going to give the digitalis [a medication that affects the heart] beforehand; I'm bringing back the other medicine called chloral hydrate that we don't use anymore because it tastes bad, and she's willing to get through the bad taste, so we're doing everything we can. This is a very different patient. —LONNY SHAVELSON, FOUNDER OF BAY AREA END OF LIFE OPTIONS, BERKELEY, CALIFORNIA

Patients themselves are not affected by how long it takes to die, because they are deeply unconscious after the first few minutes. But that's not always the case for other complications. Complications are known to have occurred in only thirty cases in Oregon as of 2017; most of the time, they involved patients regurgitating the medication. A few patients have regained consciousness, although this is very rare. It has happened in seven cases in Oregon since the law first took effect.

Law, in Washington, says she once attended the death of a young man in his thirties who had metastatic melanoma. Because he was on very high doses of pain medications, there was concern that the lethal medications might not work. "Against my better judgment, we doubled the chloral hydrate on the recommendations of an anesthesiologist," Law says. She believes the patient, who knew about the doctors' concerns, also took extra doses of a painkiller that might have added to his nausea. After ingesting the chloral hydrate, the patient immediately began to vomit, she says. "It was awful. I felt so sorry for the patient, and I felt even sorrier for the family, to watch this." She told the family she was concerned the drug might not work, the young man might wake up because he'd regurgitated so much, but he died four hours later.

"We have not had anybody *not* die," Law says of her own experiences with patients. "It may take, you know, a day— or two—but we have not had anybody that it didn't work for, which is reassuring."

ONLY ONE OF SEVERAL ROUTES TO GOOD DEATHS

The majority of medically assisted deaths are exceptionally peaceful. While Shavelson feels strongly that medically assisted deaths should be available to patients who are suffering, he doesn't think they're always the best option. "There are many, many, many ways to have a so-called good death, whatever that means to you," he says. "On June 9, 2016 [the date the aid-in-dying law took effect], we did not start having good deaths in California. We had good deaths beforehand; we have had good deaths afterwards . . . We don't have the corner on good deaths."

But medically assisted deaths are peaceful, he says. When Shavelson worked as an ER doctor earlier in his career, he witnessed traumatic deaths that he says contrast sharply with the aid-in-dying deaths he has attended. "These are not hard deaths. These are lovely deaths; these are anticipated deaths," he says. "My patients are awake and alert until the time that they die."

Just before he gives patients their prescriptions, Shavelson goes over California's nine-page report with them. Most medical professionals hate the report, he says, "but I love it. It gives me time to sit with the patient and the family."

At the end of the report, there's an optional survey. "It's questions like, 'What are the reasons you're choosing aid in dying? Are you choosing it because of a loss of autonomy?' Most of it is pretty self-evident," he says. "And then there's a little open question: 'Is there anything else?'—like an essay question, and [patients] can say whatever they want," he says.

"And the best thing I've heard in answer to the last question was, 'Tell the State thank you.'"

chapter nine
the brain and dying

WITHIN A WEEK of deciding not to start a new chemotherapy regimen, my mother was spending most of her time asleep or semiconscious. Periodically, she would wake up. Once, she requested a game of bridge, and three people pulled up chairs next to her bed for a surreal but joyful card game. At other times, she simply seemed restless. When she awoke after midnight one night, she and I toured my parents' house, peeking into rooms that had grown unfamiliar. In the dimly lit study, my husband was working on a memorial slide show. He showed it to her and she stared, unblinking, at the pictures of herself.

By the last few days, my mother was rarely conscious at all. Even when she was awake, only the most elemental parts of her were there, directing her legs to get her to the bathroom, overseeing the automated steps of brushing her teeth and wiping the sink afterward. Her mind had turned away from her daily activities, her books, her friends. Away from us—her husband, son, and two daughters. We grieved at losing her attention and presence; at the same time, we were grateful she had ceased worrying about us.

I was also deeply curious: I wanted to know where my mother's mind was. I wanted to know where *she* was.

MOST PEOPLE ARE UNCONSCIOUS
AT THE MOMENT OF DEATH

Joan Teno, the professor whose research focuses on end-of-life care and policy, says she has been troubled by similar questions about the awareness of dying patients, particularly when she talks with their families.

"I wish I had some better information to help people with that time period," she says. What she *can* tell them is that when patients' breathing patterns are starting to change and they begin actively dying, the best available evidence is that patients are not conscious or aware.

In the last weeks of life, consciousness tends to ebb and flow. Dying patients may be unconscious for hours, semi-aware at other times, and completely alert at others. But by the time they reach their final few hours, most people with a fatal disease are not fully conscious. In a 1998 study of patients with terminal cancer, researchers found that 79 percent were awake and alert two weeks before death. But the number dropped to 32 percent in the last two days of life, and as people neared the moment of death, that number continued to fall. Studies have found that only a minority of dying patients, somewhere between 8 and 30 percent, remain conscious until the very end of life.

This gradual loss of consciousness has two main causes: First, medications that are prescribed to treat pain and other symptoms can also affect consciousness. Second, as the rest of the body dies, the brain itself begins to fail.

A SIDE EFFECT OF PAIN TREATMENTS

Most dying people in developed nations are given opioids to control pain or dyspnea, and these medications often make patients less alert. Even when a particular drug doesn't affect a person's mental state, it may do so in combinations with other drugs, and dying patients are usually on multiple medications.

But it's not easy to measure just how much the drugs contribute to this lack of awareness. Opioids, for instance, usually make people drowsy or less conscious in the first day or two after they're administered, but patients quickly develop a tolerance to this effect. In one study, cancer patients with a significant increase in doses of opioids showed a corresponding increase in cognitive impairment, but that impairment disappeared a week later. Furthermore, there are even times when drugs make people *more* alert because they treat pain that might otherwise reduce mental function.

When researchers have tested advanced cancer patients who are not on opioids, they've found many of these patients are less alert and have poorer cognitive functioning than healthy people. The tests underline what neurologists already know: Opioids and other drugs are not the only factor in dying patients' gradual loss of awareness.

WHEN YOU'RE DYING, YOUR BRAIN IS ALSO SHUTTING DOWN

What happens to your brain as you die depends on your disease or condition, but dying changes your body chemistry, and that affects your brain, says James Bernat, a Dartmouth neurologist and leading authority on the issue of brain death. For example, if you have end-stage metastatic cancer, you usually stop drinking fluids, which causes you to become dehydrated. That, in turn, leads to low blood pressure. The condition will probably also interfere with your electrolyte balance, sodium levels, and chloride levels.

"The brain cells are exquisitely sensitive," Bernat says. To function, neurons require a specialized environment: the right temperature, the right amount of oxygen, the right amount of glucose. Even an interruption of twenty seconds in the supply of glycogen and oxygen can affect how well the brain works. "The brain doesn't store anything, any fuel, so interruptions of oxygen and glucose cause rather immediate impairments of the brain," Bernat explains.

The best model for what's going on in the brain close to death is a condition called *metabolic encephalopathy,* which means the chemistry of the brain as a whole is somehow disturbed. This damage to the brain may affect vision and hearing, it may produce tremors and weakness, it may affect thinking and consciousness. "It's common for people to slow down, to sleep a lot, to become unconscious in addition to sleep," Bernat says. "And that's the result of this metabolic derangement within the brain cells caused by the changes that occur during dying."

As a person's brain breaks down, individual neurons all over the organ are affected, so it's hard to determine exactly which parts will be most impacted. Neurologists do know that the most resilient brain cells are those that developed earlier in human evolution, such as those in the brainstem. These parts of the brain are evolutionarily ancient, Bernat says: "If you look at a human brainstem and an alligator brainstem, they're relatively similar." Cells in the brainstem—the part of the brain that helps keep you awake—are especially resistant to the damaging effects of a fatal disease. But even when those cells are working, a person may not be conscious.

The cells that have developed most recently in human evolution are much more susceptible to a loss of glycogen and oxygen. Those include cells in the cerebral hemispheres and the hippocampus, the parts of your brain that make you aware of your subjective experience. Because metabolic encephalopathy affects those parts of the brain first and most drastically, most dying patients gradually lose consciousness while other parts of their brains—the parts that make it possible for them to breathe or for their hearts to beat, for instance—continue to function.

WAKEFULNESS AND AWARENESS

For years, neurologists have divided consciousness into these two dimensions: wakefulness and awareness. You can have one without the other, but you need both in order to be conscious. For instance, people in a coma are neither awake nor aware. In contrast, people in other states may be aware but not awake—when they're asleep and dreaming. Patients in a vegetative state are awake but not aware. Their eyes may open every day for a period of wakefulness, and then shut during sleep at night. But they have no sense of self and environment, no thoughts. They don't have subjective experiences. In some sense, these people are "gone," at least temporarily. They're not aware.

If doctors suspect there's something wrong, they try to determine whether a person is conscious at all. If a patient's eyes are open, they can ask him questions. If the person is unable to respond verbally, he can signal with head movements, gestures, or eye movements. Even if his eyes are closed, neurologists can use a series of bedside tests. They ask a patient to stick out his tongue, to touch his nose, to kick an object, to take the medical professional's hand. They make a loud noise and watch to see if the patient's eyelids flutter in response.

If patients are still unresponsive, determining whether they're conscious becomes more difficult. When a patient is dying and has slipped into a state of semi-consciousness or unconsciousness, "we can't know the extent to which the patient is aware because they make relatively few responses and we rely on responses as an indication of awareness," Bernat says. "We can't get into their mind and see what's going on in there, to experience what they experience. So we infer the quality of their conscious life as a result of what responses they make to our stimuli. And if they're not making many responses, and we really don't know exactly what's going on, we assume that they're unconscious."

There are also states along the continuum of wakefulness and awareness in which people are partly awake, or partly aware—the kind of consciousness that a dying patient might experience before dropping into a state of full unconsciousness. In 2002, researchers came up with an official name for a relatively new category of patients with severe brain damage whose behavior was inconsistent: the minimally conscious state, or MCS. Unlike people in a vegetative state, these patients sometimes show definite evidence of awareness.

The problem is that it's very difficult to distinguish between the two—to determine whether an unresponsive patient is wakeful but completely unaware, or still retains at least some degree of awareness.

SEEING INSIDE OTHER PEOPLE'S MINDS

In the past few years, neurologists have made significant breakthroughs, and they're starting to see glimmers on the horizon, hints that someday they might be able to communicate with unconscious or unresponsive patients, says David Hovda, director of the UCLA Brain Injury Research Center. "The technology that we're able to use now, that we couldn't use five years ago, is so remarkable that we are now beginning, just beginning, to be able to communicate to the brain, and to people that were in a coma," Hovda says.

That's exactly what happened in a now-famous neurological study in 2010 that Hovda sent me—"we didn't publish it; I wish to God I had," he says. In the study, Adrian Owen, Steven Laureys, and six other researchers tried new ways of testing for responses in fifty-four comatose patients who had severe brain injuries. Twenty-three of the patients' brain disorders were especially severe: They had been diagnosed as being in a vegetative state, of "wakefulness but not awareness," although neurologists later concluded that some of them had been misdiagnosed.

In my favorite part of the experiment, the patients were placed in a functional MRI scanner and told to visualize two different activities, with thirty-second rests between them. In the first activity, they were told to imagine they were swinging a tennis racquet to hit a tennis ball back and forth with an instructor for thirty-second periods, punctuated by periods of rest. In the second activity, patients were asked to imagine walking from room to room in their homes or along the streets of a familiar city, visualizing what they'd be likely to see in their wanderings.

For five of the patients—four of whom had been diagnosed as in a vegetative state—the results were remarkable. The motor cortex, the center in the brain where signals both for actual physical activities and imagined ones originate, fired at the appropriate times. Evidently, these patients were imagining playing tennis when cued, and were able to imagine stopping the exercise when they were supposed to rest. In four of the patients, the parts of the brain associated with spatial imagery fired when they were being asked to imagine the spatial task of walking around their homes or a city.

The researchers tried an additional experiment for one patient and a control group: Each person was placed in an fMRI scan and asked several questions that were easy to verify—questions such as, "Is your father's name Alexander?" They were told to imagine one of the activities to say "yes," and the other to say "no." The patient "answered" five out of six questions correctly, in each case, imagining the activity that corresponded with the correct answer to the question.

The authors were cautious not to overstate the implications of their study. The fact that a person's brain revealed activity in response to a request during the experiment doesn't reveal how much that brain was responding at other times. However, for at least five of the patients, the answer to the question of whether the person's mind was still aware and functioning at all, was an emphatic *yes*. And until doctors used the functional MRI to check, they had been unable to determine that these patients were at least partly aware.

Since the tennis experiment, researchers have continued to learn more about patients in a minimally conscious state, or what is now also called "covert consciousness," in which doctors can't detect consciousness through standard bedside exams. One study found that when minimally conscious patients hear their own names, their brains respond, although more slowly than healthy brains do. Other studies suggest these patients are at least partly aware: They seem to retain some language recognition, for instance, and feel pain.

Still, there is much that researchers don't know about patients who are in a minimally conscious state—a condition Bernat believes should really be called the minimally responsive state because some of these patients' consciousness might even be normal. "What we know is that [the patients] don't make a lot of responses," he says. "We don't know the extent to which they're conscious because we can't really test it directly." It's also hard to determine what any of these patients are feeling, or what this experience between full consciousness and unconsciousness might be like.

CONSCIOUSNESS ISN'T LIKE FLIPPING A SWITCH

Human awareness is very sophisticated, and neurologists don't ultimately understand how it works. Even when you're fully conscious and able to communicate, that feeling—the subjective experience in normal consciousness—is extremely complex, says Caroline Schnakers, a neurologist who has worked with minimally conscious and vegetative state patients. Imagine you go to a restaurant, and later want to describe your experience to friends. That involves attention, working memory, and long-term memory in your brain, she explains. It requires visual and auditory perception and olfactory processing of the experience. As you eat and chat with your dining companions, your brain has to process how you feel emotionally about the food and conversation. It has to compute that the restaurant meal is important enough to you to relate to your friends, so you employ metacognition, which allows you to observe yourself and your experience.

That's all just to remember a simple restaurant meal when your consciousness is functioning normally. Understanding the processes at work for patients with disorders of consciousness is even more difficult. One of the thorny questions in the experiments with these patients is whether they are necessarily aware when their brains respond, Bernat says. For the tennis-imaging study, researchers proved that when patients' brains were registering responses, their awareness was, too—the fact that a patient could answer the yes-or-no questions showed that he was conscious of what his brain was experiencing. But that's not always easy to demonstrate. Bernat gives the example of a condition called face blindness or prosopagnosia, in which people lose the ability to recognize familiar faces. They can see the parts—the eyes, nose, ears, and mouth—but they can't put those parts together as a whole to recognize who a person is. In a study testing people with this condition, researchers showed patients photographs of famous people's faces. They asked the patients about the photos, and at the same time monitored physical responses such as their heart rates, respiratory rates, and temperatures.

Patients told researchers they didn't recognize the faces,

but the monitors indicated something else: The photos of familiar faces were registering significantly differently from those of strangers. The monitors revealed that even though the patients weren't aware of it, their brains *did* recognize familiar faces on some levels. "Even though the person wasn't aware, something in their brains was registering it. Isn't that interesting?" Bernat marvels. "It just proves to us that awareness is a pretty complicated phenomenon. It's not a simple flip-a-switch phenomenon."

THE IMPLICATIONS FOR DYING PEOPLE

Researching what consciousness feels like for people close to death can be especially problematic. "What do we know about the experience that the dying patient has?" Bernat asks. "There isn't much out there. It hasn't been really studied." Even if doctors could estimate better when a person is very close to death, most patients—or their families—would object to having electrodes attached to their heads in their last few hours.

But when people are very close to death and are no longer responding, that state of consciousness is generally considered a coma, Schnakers says. Unlike minimally conscious people, who are emerging from a coma, these patients are entering one. "And when you are in a coma, you should not be able to feel anything. So you should not perceive sounds around you; you should not have any experience complex enough that you can remember it." When coma patients have been placed in a scanner, there is very little brain activity, she says. Even the brain of a person in normal sleep shows more activity than these patients because the sleepers are capable of dreaming. As far as neurologists can tell, coma patients don't have subjective experiences at all.

But what about before then, before a dying patient falls

into a final coma? What if unresponsive dying patients, like patients in a minimally conscious state, are sometimes still aware rather than unconscious?

The most relevant lesson neuroscientists' studies with minimally conscious patients have for understanding the consciousness of dying people is that dying patients may be more aware than doctors usually think, Bernat believes: "My take on it is that dying people have higher degrees of awareness than they're often given credit for." It's possible that dying people in this semiconscious state might still be thinking, or dreaming, or experiencing some type of confused, partial awareness.

But Bernat and other neurologists advise caution in applying the results of studies like the tennis-imaging experiment to dying people. The consciousness of a dying person is not identical to that of an MCS patient, Bernat says. And the vegetative state and the various MCS states are more like rough categories than pure diagnoses: "They can be very, very different from each other in terms of the areas of the brain involved, the severity, the cause and many other factors." For instance, a minimally conscious state might be caused by a traumatic brain injury, an intracranial hemorrhage, neuronal damage from lack of oxygen and blood flow during cardiac arrest, or encephalitis. "They all can yield clinical syndromes that resemble each other even though they're caused by different things," he says. "So, it's a bit of a mess."

Even one particular minimally conscious person may be far more self-aware, far more often, than another. Awareness in minimally conscious patients may be intermittent, it may be partial, or it may only appear in response to certain stimuli, he says.

Just as they do in patients in minimally conscious states, the conscious states of dying people vary significantly, depending on factors such as how fast the brain deteriorates in comparison to the rest of the body, and how much a particular person's brain breaks down—how severe the metabolic encephalopathy is—before she dies. "There is a range of severity of metabolic encephalopathies, where mild forms of it can produce just a little bit of confusion, slowness of thinking, slowness of response," Bernat says.

A STATE OF CONFUSION

There is another model for thinking about what happens in a dying person's brain. When metabolic encephalopathy occurs in dying patients, the name is often used interchangeably with another, more familiar term: delirium. The medical field has only recently started understanding that delirium is a serious problem, says Marian Grant, the hospice and palliative care nurse practitioner: "It's a sign of brain dysfunction—something is causing a change in the level of consciousness." The symptoms of delirium can mimic those of dementia, but delirium tends to happen fast, over the course of a few hours or a couple of days. Patients lose their ability to focus, and they may lose awareness of their environment. Delirious patients don't think clearly—their consciousness is clouded. They're usually confused and disoriented, and they may have trouble remembering words, reading, writing, or understanding what other people are saying. In one kind of delirium, they become very restless. In a second kind, they withdraw and lapse into lethargy.

Most metabolic encephalopathies produce delirium, but there are other causes as well: drug intoxication and withdrawal, poisoning, and psychiatric disorders. One of the most common causes is the dying process, and as many as 60 to 88 percent of hospice patients may experience delirium at some point. The condition is often a sign that a patient is moving into the last days of life.

"Now, is that the electrolyte abnormalities that come with dying?" Grant asks. "Is that the body breaking down in ways that affect the brain? Is that the result of prolonged lower levels of oxygen? I don't think we have a good explanation. But I have seen it often in the hospital; I've seen it often in hospice, and I usually think, 'She has maybe only a few days left.'"

In a study of 154 cancer patients who had at least one episode of delirium, the psychiatrist William Breitbart and his colleagues set out to gather evidence about what that experience was like. Most of the patients received treatment with the antipsychotic olanzapine and fully recovered from their delirium, although fifty-three of the patients died before the study was completed. About half the patients who recovered remembered their delirium experience. The patients reported that while they were in the midst of their delirium, they could hear relatives and staff talking, and later, some remembered other experiences, including hallucinations. For 80 percent of the patients who remembered it, the experience was distressing, mostly because of frightening hallucinations or delusions, Breitbart and his colleagues write.

But the condition and its effects are not easy to pigeonhole. "Delirium by its nature waxes and wanes," Grant explains. "So people are lucid one minute, and then not lucid moments later, which is part of the challenge to assessing it and to managing it." When she worked in hospice, Grant says she often needed to educate families about the effects of delirium "because, all of a sudden, Grandma was raving like a sailor, or she was seeing things, and she had never hallucinated before. And this is very distressing to the family."

Delirium can range from mild to very severe. It also behaves in different ways and can result in a wide array of symptoms affecting patients' alertness and cognitive functions. There are two main kinds: hyperactive and hypoactive. Hypoactive patients have low energy and are usually less aware; Grant says she jokes that these are the patients that medical staff often call "good patients," because they lie quietly in their beds, not causing any trouble for busy nurses. But their condition still needs to be assessed and perhaps treated, she says. In contrast, hyperactive delirium fits the popular image. These patients tend to be restless, and they are more likely to experience hallucinations or delusions.

The hyperactive condition is also sometimes called terminal restlessness or terminal agitation because some patients become extremely agitated. They may try to get out of bed or pull their clothes off. When Grant's elderly father-in-law broke his hip and was close to death, he was delirious and couldn't remember that his hip was broken. "He kept trying to get out of bed," Grant says. "It was tragic, because he just didn't get it. And in the hospital, all they could do was tie him down, and he didn't understand why he was tied down; that made him even more agitated."

Despite her father-in-law's turmoil, Grant says that in her personal clinical experience, delirium doesn't seem to be distressing to patients. "They are distressed in the moment because they don't get what's going on," she says. But "when they say they are seeing people from the past, or they see angels at the foot of the bed, I have no idea what's really going on, but they don't seem discomforted by that."

In fact, these patients often find their hallucinations or visions comforting. "They are not frightened by the fact that they see people who are former loved ones who are no longer living," Grant says.

THE DREAMS OF DYING PEOPLE

"Most people dying a slow death will have a significant period of confusion before death," says the palliative care expert James Hallenbeck. His students often find the prospect of losing their sanity, their grounding in reality, terrifying. When he talks with students about this, he asks them: "Why does that scare you? Every night, you're absolutely bat-shit crazy while you're dreaming. It's not the *dreaming* that's the problem, it's whether it's a good dream or a bad dream."

During our nightly dreams, he points out, "we're all certifiably insane. And fortunately, we're paralyzed so we don't hurt anybody while we're flying like Superman or whatever we're doing. It's the content that matters, not the confusion." Researchers like Breitbart have found that delirium is a real illness, and it's one that's treatable. But the research and experience of many palliative care workers also points to patients who have positive feelings as their minds drift away from reality. It seems likely that the dreamy states and confusion of so many dying people might be both positive and negative, in the same way that we have both nightmares and good dreams during normal sleep.

In her last couple of weeks, when my mother's mind seemed to be floating off somewhere else most of the time, she would sometimes raise her arms in the air, plucking at invisible objects with her fingers. I didn't know then that this sort of picking at objects is common in dying people.

Once, I captured her hands in mine and asked what she'd been doing. "Putting things away," she answered, smiling dreamily.

What are the dream states of dying people? Hallenbeck would like to see neurologists monitor their brain waves: "My theory is that there would be wave forms suggestive of sleep superimposed on wave forms suggestive of wakefulness. That is, the normal 'firewall' between waking and dreaming consciousness breaks down."

Whatever else that semi–dream state of the dying may be, it's usually pleasant for most people, Hallenbeck says. "My mother, the day she died, she had all of her animals do a parade before her and was happy as a clam. That kind of thing is incredibly common, and transcultural."

The actual content of the visions may depend on a person's particular background and experiences, however. Some people may see angels, complete with feathered wings and halos. At the Veterans Administration hospice in Palo Alto, where Hallenbeck is a doctor, one patient with a fatal disease had a travel vision. Instead of an angel at the gate, he saw a military guard at the door who told him, "Go back, sir. It's not your time to deploy."

Hallenbeck says these visions are different from the near-death experiences some people report, the ones that involve the classic sensation of going toward a light or through a tunnel. The visions are more likely to be interwoven with waking reality. For instance, patients will tell nurses or family visitors, "Don't sit there—there's a baby in the chair," he says. Or they'll ask, "Who was that kid who walked past there?"

In the most common visions he's witnessed, patients see deceased relatives. He thinks of the experiences as completing a circle of birth and death in patients' minds.

Traditional medical systems, and even hospice, underestimate the prevalence of these experiences for dying patients, Hallenbeck says, "because, while they're in that limbic state of confusion, they usually know enough to know it's a bad idea to tell doctors about it." Once, Hallenbeck noticed a patient's daughter reading *Guided by the Light: Following Your Angelic Guides*, and he asked if she was trying to figure out what would happen to her father when he died. "She said, 'No, Dad's room has been chock-full of dead relatives for the last two months, and I'm trying to figure out what the hell they're doing there.'" Hallenbeck had visited the patient every day for two months, and the patient had never mentioned seeing deceased family members.

Hallenbeck has learned to look for clues. "If they're looking a little fuzzy-headed, I'll look at their eyes and I've learned to ask, 'What did you see?'" If he pushes, patients will sometimes acknowledge a vision: "Well, you just won't believe it, my dead grandmother sitting up there." But they often don't.

Researchers led by Dr. Christopher Kerr at a hospice center outside Buffalo, New York, have been studying dying people's dreams, and they also believe that family and medical staff may sometimes fail to take dreams seriously, in part because so many dying people move in and out of delirium. One feature of this research team's work stands out: They've been interviewing the *patients,* rather than just family members.

Most of the patients interviewed, 88 percent, had at least one dream or vision. And those dreams usually felt different to them from normal dreams. For one thing, the dreams seemed clearer and more real. The dying patients' dreams were more intense, and for many, felt the same as the times when they were awake, according to an article about the study in the *Journal of Palliative Medicine.*

And what did they dream about? Seventy-two percent dreamed about reuniting with people who had already died. Fifty-nine percent said they dreamed about getting ready to travel somewhere. Twenty-eight percent dreamed about meaningful experiences in the past. (The researchers interviewed their patients every day until the patients died or could no longer talk to them, so the same individuals often reported dreams about multiple subjects.)

Based on his research and work with patients, Breitbart believes that these dreams are the hallucinations that accompany delirium. But the Buffalo researchers theorize that these dreams are different from hallucinations or delirium. Delirious or confused patients tend to have disorganized thinking, to be anxious or agitated, to be confused about their surroundings, they note. While some of the patients interviewed for the study were delirious at times, the researchers write that they were clearheaded when describing their dreams. The Buffalo study finds that the dreams were comforting, positive experiences. That's also what Fred Schwartz, the medical director of Hospice New York, has observed about patients who believe they are seeing and conversing with deceased family members. He says the visions are very real to the patients, and they are almost always a positive experience: "When they have these events happen to them, they are so relieved, happy, joyful—any fear that they've had is dissipated." After the visions, patients are usually ecstatic, he says. He remembers sitting at the bedside of a dying patient who told him her brother was in the room. It was the happiest he'd seen her in her two years in hospice.

While the visions often involve family members who have died, sometimes they are about other subjects or people. One dying patient's description of how happy he was at seeing an angel surrounded by light and beauty left the hospice team in tears, Schwartz says. And because the patient was able to articulate his happiness, his description served as a gift to his caregiver and hospice team. "It's a gift, because, you know, we all have to die, and we all have the same fears about what is it going to be like for me or my family members when this happens—an experience like that is very powerful," Schwartz says.

SO WAS MY MOTHER CONSCIOUS
WHEN SHE WAS DYING?

For much of my mother's last three weeks of life, I felt a similar sense of having received a gift because so much of the experience was filled with meaning and family closeness. But as far as I know, there were no conversations with long-lost relatives or wonderful visions. I do know she experienced difficulties, and that she suffered.

"You understand that not everybody goes gentle into that good night, right?" warns Judith Schwarz. Just as consciousness tends to wax and wane, so does any sense of peace for even many of the easier deaths. My mother's state of consciousness in her last week seems to best match Breitbart's description of hypoactive delirium, in which a patient feels a loss of energy and gradually enters a coma as the brain deteriorates.

That still doesn't mean her consciousness was completely gone in her last couple of days. After decades of observing patients with traumatic brain injuries, neurologists have learned something about the mechanics of what happens as the brain breaks down. And in recent years, new technologies have brought insights into the experiences of semiconscious patients. But despite the leaps forward in recent knowledge, models of consciousness remain primitive, James Bernat emphasizes. Research still hasn't found a way to "understand how this lump of white and gray matter in the brain that weighs three pounds, leads us to be able to appreciate Mozart and the color red and many other things."

Realizing the limits of what we understand about the brain has made Bernat humble. "One thing that I have learned as a neurologist interested in coma and vegetative state and disorders of consciousness is that if we clinicians make an error assessing the level of awareness of someone, it's usually in the direction of saying they're unaware when they are actually aware, and not in the other direction," he says.

Neuroscientist Jimo Borjigin says something similar: "We don't understand the dying process of the brain." When she studied the subject, "the more I researched, the more I realized that we know so little about the dying brain, the dying process," she says. "Even though it happens to every single one of us, we know almost nothing."

Judith Schwarz told me that when her own mother died, she also spent most of the time drifting through semiconscious or sleeping states. "And I was very conscious of the fact, the day before she died, that if I spoke to her, I was pulling her back from some place—I was very conscious of that, that she was someplace else that was comfortable for her," Schwarz says. "And when I would ask her a question she would have to struggle to come back to answer it.

"So I stopped doing that."

chapter ten
the last few hours

DYING OFTEN HAS a final phase, the time when a person starts a rapidly deepening decline. During this slide in the last two or three days of life, when people become too weak to cough or swallow, some start to make a noise in the backs of their throats. The sound—sometimes "like a purring of a cat," James Hallenbeck says—can be deeply disturbing for those who witness it, as if the patient is suffering severe pain.

That's not what it feels like to the person dying, as far as anyone can tell. In fact, doctors and nurses believe that the phenomenon—which is commonly called a death rattle—probably doesn't hurt. "It's bothersome to everybody else usually, but almost never to the [dying] person," Hallenbeck says.

A growing body of research is shedding light on the signs and symptoms of approaching death, patients' experiences, and the science behind near-death experiences and what those may tell us about the process of dying.

While these insights are tantalizing, they also underline the limits of our knowledge. The very way we talk about death often describes what witnesses see, rather than what dying people experience. "We speak of 'death agonies,' even though the dying person is too far gone to be aware of them, and even though much of what occurs is due simply to muscle spasm induced by the blood's terminal acidity," Sherwin Nuland writes in his book, *How We Die.*

In the research about what happens when we die, it's this distinction between what the people around a dying person—family, friends, medical professionals—see and experience, and what a dying person actually feels, that remains shrouded in mystery.

What do we really know about the experience of dying patients in those final days?

DETERMINING WHEN ACTIVE DYING STARTS IS EASY—IN HINDSIGHT

In the last two weeks of her life, my mother was ready and eager to die. Her chemotherapy had stopped working and her body was shutting down. At one point, she asked a hospice nurse how much time she had remaining. The nurse, no doubt from a sense of compassion, gave my mother an estimate: maybe three days.

Three days passed. And then four, and then five.

I have a vivid memory of my mother staring at the mirror after I had helped her to the bathroom. She had been brushing her teeth, but she paused, studying her own reflection, seeing and not-seeing. "It's so unfair," she said. "It was so unfair of that nurse to say I had three days left." My mother, who did not criticize nurses or doctors or complain about her illness, had been pitched off balance by an inaccurate prognosis.

In healthier times, she would have realized it was probably her question that was unfair. While doctors can usually tell that someone is dying, it's tough to accurately guess the day or hour of death ahead of time. In fact, studies have shown they tend to get it wrong about 80 percent of the time, mostly

by being overly optimistic. "We don't have a crystal ball," says
Michelle Appenzeller, the clinical director at Durango's Hospice of Mercy.

> *When do people die? I have had patients hang on in
> situations that make no physiologic sense. They should
> have been dead days ago. I had a guy in hospice who
> had a 105-degree temperature. He was septic; he had a
> systemic infection. He was in my hospice; we were not
> giving him fluids; we were not doing anything. But the
> patient was originally from Asia, and a family member
> was on the way to say good-bye to him. He hung in there
> until that family member got off the plane. I could not
> explain it. I've had little old ladies who haven't had
> anything to eat or drink for two or three weeks who live
> on. They're not awake, but they're just lingering. Are
> they waiting for someone? Is it not time? Do they want
> the family not to be there?* —MARIAN GRANT, HOSPICE AND
> PALLIATIVE CARE NURSE PRACTITIONER

When nurses and doctors say a dying patient is "active" or
"actively dying," they usually mean the person is in the last
days or hours of life. But the term presupposes that medical
professionals can determine when those last hours or days
are.

Based on sharp changes in symptoms, hospice staff members can often tell patients or their caregivers roughly when to
expect death. "We can *kind of* know," Appenzeller says. After
experiencing a steady, aggressive decline in the last week, you
tend to become much less responsive in your last two days.
Your symptoms intensify. Your body begins to give up less
crucial functions in order to preserve your heart and your
brain. You start to feel drowsier and more fatigued, growing
significantly weaker and staying in bed more. Your muscular

functions rapidly begin to degenerate, and your heart's pumping rhythm becomes feebler, which means your body is sending less blood to your kidneys. Then your kidneys and other organs start to fail.

While people who work with the dying recognize the general signs, the period of active dying can still be difficult-to-impossible to identify precisely. "I've heard the nurses say, 'They're actively dying,'—and I've heard [them say] that for weeks," Appenzeller says. "Nobody's really actively dying for weeks."

David Hui, the palliative care specialist, wondered if there was a way to be more scientific in making those predictions. So he and his colleagues combed through research literature that mentioned signs of approaching death and then talked with palliative care doctors and nurses. For their first study, they ended up with a list of ten signs to monitor in dying patients.

What they learned in this study, and a later one that examined even more signs, was both enlightening and unsatisfying: The signs that patients are most likely to exhibit tend to be the least dependable in predicting whether death is imminent. But the researchers discovered that if a patient has one or more of thirteen signs—ranging from a death rattle, to irregular breathing patterns, to decreased responsiveness to visual stimuli—there's a very strong chance the person is within three days of dying. And the signs in combination are even more reliable as indicators of whether someone is about to die. If a patient is still walking around, if his organs are functioning reasonably well, and if his face appears relatively normal, doctors can be pretty confident he won't die in the next three days, Hui says. But if a patient is bedbound and unconscious and the crease between his cheek and nose—the nasolabial fold—starts to disappear, it's likely he will die within hours or days.

The problem is that the list of signs isn't foolproof. A patient may have the irregular breathing patterns associated with being close to death but still linger for weeks. Or patients may die without ever exhibiting these signs. Even the model distinguishing between patients who are walking around and functional, and those who are unconscious and bedbound, doesn't help much for the patients who fall somewhere in the middle, Hui says. These patients may have a 40 percent chance of dying in their next three days, and that's not enough to predict the day of death with any confidence.

It's also important to remember the difference between *signs,* which outsiders can observe, and *symptoms,* which the patient experiences, Hui says. For instance, while both Cheyne-Stokes breathing and dyspnea can be associated with dying, the first is a sign and the second, a symptom.

A SYMPTOM IS SOMETHING THE PATIENT EXPERIENCES; A SIGN IS SOMETHING DOCTORS OBSERVE

Cheyne-Stokes breathing, named after two doctors who first described it in detail, is a cycle of breathing patterns. The dying person starts to take deeper and faster breaths, her breathing rising in a crescendo. Next, breaths become slower and shallower until they stop altogether, sometimes for a frighteningly long period. Then the pattern starts over again. A terminally ill person with Cheyne-Stokes breathing is very likely within hours or days of dying, although the pattern can sometimes show up in other, nonterminal, conditions (in which case it's not a sign that the patient is dying).

Like the death rattle, Cheyne-Stokes can be difficult for a patient's family to watch. The dying person may seem to be struggling for each breath, drowning from lack of air. But that's not what Cheyne-Stokes is like for the patient. Medical professionals are pretty certain the experience isn't painful, or even distressing. Cheyne-Stokes breathing is usually quite slow, "and the slower the breathing, the less likely the patient's having distress," says Margaret Campbell, the palliative care pioneer and professor of nursing. "Rapid breathing goes along with distress; slow breathing does not." Furthermore, by the time patients exhibit Cheyne-Stokes breathing, they're almost always unconscious.

In contrast, dyspnea is, by definition, a subjective experience. *Air hunger*, it's often called, or simply *breathlessness*. It's the feeling of having difficulty breathing, and it's a symptom of approaching death, although not everyone who experiences this is dying. Hui describes the feeling as being as if, "'I can't get enough air inside my body.'"

The intensity varies, but dyspnea can be very uncomfortable, says Mac Johnson, an internist in Durango, Colorado. "If you've ever been underwater and can't get your breath—it's the same feeling." It's treatable, most commonly with opioids, but also with techniques such as elevating patients' heads, training patients to control their breathing, or simply opening windows or turning on a fan to increase the flow of air.

Dyspnea may be caused by any one of several different phenomena, and it can be made worse by anxiety. Patients may have an obstruction in the airways or lungs, or their lungs may be stiff or injured, so they have to work harder to breathe. They may have weak respiratory muscles or a weak heart because of an illness or aging. Or a patient's nervous system may be damaged, so her body has less drive to breathe.

Only patients can say whether they feel short of breath, and therefore only conscious patients can experience the condition. But they can be conscious and no longer able to respond: "Most people, when they're very close to passing, can no longer tell us what they're experiencing," Campbell says. If these patients experience shortness of breath, it may sometimes go untreated. "We can't ask them, 'Are you uncomfortable?'" Busy nurses without a lot of experience in tending to dying people might easily miss the symptoms. In her clinical practice, Campbell would sometimes find a non-communicative patient in respiratory distress, despite having left instructions for treating the condition if it occurred. "So I would find the nurse and I'd say, 'Your patient is in respiratory distress.' And he or she would say, 'Really?'"

FIGURING OUT WHAT PATIENTS ARE ACTUALLY EXPERIENCING

In her work as a researcher, Campbell has been especially interested in this difference between what witnesses think patients experience and what patients actually feel. That was what first led her to study the death rattle. "For years and years and years, I took care of people who were very close to passing, and noticed some made noise, and some didn't," she says. "And over time I noticed that while the patient was making noise, the patient didn't seem to be in any distress."

Somewhere between 35 and 50 percent of dying patients produce a death rattle in the last day or two of life, which happens when patients are too weak or unconscious to clear secretions at the backs of their throats. Since patients also didn't exhibit any signs of discomfort when they made the sound, Campbell deduced that they weren't in pain—the same conclusion most other nurses and doctors have reached. So, she was surprised that doctors continued to treat the death rattle with medications that had potential side effects such as dry mouth, urinary retention, and confusion.

Campbell decided to conduct a study, examining and recording the differences between dying patients who had the death rattle and those who did not. Based on that study of seventy-one people, she concluded that the death rattle generally does not cause discomfort or pain for patients—although it often does for family members or even medical professionals who witness it. "We may want to acknowledge that death can be a messy experience characterized by incontinence, odors, and sometimes noisy breathing," Campbell writes. "The mess, fuss, and noise associated with birth are not viewed negatively, in fact they are normalized. Must we attempt to 'sanitize' with medications the noise that may occur during dying?"

The situation is even worse for patients who can't communicate their suffering. People experienced in working with the dying can usually figure out whether those patients feel shortness of breath, even if the patients can't tell them, Campbell says. Instead of relying on their diaphragms to breathe, these patients may use accessory muscles. They sometimes make a guttural grunting sound. They sometimes have paradoxical breathing. "With normal resting breathing, your chest and abdomen move in the same direction at the same time," explains Campbell, "but with difficult breathing, there's a paradox and the abdomen is going in when the chest is going out and vice versa."

It usually takes experience to recognize this group of signs of discomfort, and time to observe them closely, both of which may be missing in the hectic atmosphere of many hospitals. So Campbell did a study of signs of shortness of breath in patients who couldn't report it themselves, and she developed a scale for measuring respiratory distress—the Respiratory Distress Observation Scale, or RDOS. The scale is being adopted in more and more hospices, she says, and it's likely more patients are much more comfortable as a result.

Shortness of breath, Cheyne-Stokes breathing, and the death rattle are a small subset of the struggles dying people may experience with daily functions that are usually taken for granted. "We don't even need to think about breathing normally and that's because it's all such a fundamental function, that our very primitive brain—the brainstem—regulates that part," Hui says.

PAIN IN THE LAST DAYS OF LIFE

Just as Campbell created a scale to measure respiratory distress in patients who couldn't communicate, other researchers are developing similar scales to measure pain in these patients. "Pain is a little bit easier to detect because it's all in the face, and it's an ouch face," Campbell says. If unnecessary invasive procedures are avoided, she says, most dying patients seem to be comfortable in their final hours: "If we're letting them die naturally, then they're most likely going to be comfortable during those last hours."

Cicely Saunders, the modern hospice pioneer, observes that pain usually seemed to disappear right at the end of a person's life: The actual process of dying "is almost always painless and peaceful," she writes. "Mental and physical pain usually recede during the few days before death and certainly in the last hours."

Numerous studies support Saunders's professional observations, according to a 2005 review of other studies by William Plonk and Robert Arnold. Plonk and Arnold cite one study that found pain among patients dying at home peaked about a month before they died. No one is sure why pain might decrease right at the end of life. Maybe it's ketosis, a side effect of the body's using up glucose reserves, or uremia, or a buildup of endorphins, but no conclusive studies have determined the cause.

While most patients are peaceful at the moment of death, it's important to remember that the final days leading up to that moment can be punishing, according to researchers in a 1990 New Zealand study. The researchers found that 36 percent of patients experienced at least some difficulties in their last two days of life, including pain, shortness of breath, restlessness and agitation, incontinence or, for a small percentage, nausea and vomiting. By the time these patients reached their last forty-eight hours, 64 percent were peaceful—and that number reached 91.5 percent at the time of death. "Patients certainly do die peacefully, but the final days may be difficult for the patient, the family, and the caregivers," the researchers caution.

Many of the symptoms that appear in the very last days of life are caused by multi-organ failure, leading to a general metabolic disorder, they conclude. As people enter the last days or hours of life, entire systems in their bodies begin to disintegrate.

"If you think about what really happens to patients when they are entering the last hours or days of life, eventually it's a loss of the neurocognitive [functions]," Hui agrees. As the brain starts to fail, that failure affects the rest of the body's systems.

THE WAY THE BODY BREAKS DOWN

We don't usually die organ by organ, Hallenbeck says. Instead, it's a "very organic, analogue-y" process: "For anything other than a sudden death, it's this falling apart of a whole lot of checks and balances that we have in our body that are—even for doctors—out of sight and out of mind."

For instance, when your respiratory system is functioning normally, carbon dioxide levels stimulate it to adjust automatically to different conditions. When the amount of carbon dioxide in your system rises, your body reacts by breathing harder. When the amount drops, your breathing slows down. But as your brain breaks down, it begins to let go of its role in maintaining this balance. And when it does, your system overreacts. You breathe too hard when the carbon dioxide level goes up and you stop breathing altogether for a few seconds when it goes down. That's Cheyne-Stokes, Hallenbeck says.

He gives another example: When you're healthy, your capillaries automatically release the appropriate amounts of blood into your tissues. Most people don't give the process any thought, but it's actually quite complex. "You want to let some blood through, but not too much," he says. "If it's too much, then your blood pressure disappears, and if it's not enough, your tissues aren't alive." This systemic action starts malfunctioning when people are close to death. Doctors can detect the results in mottled areas that appear on patients' legs or upper arms, patches of skin that turn mostly red, with a little bluish and white coloring. This is different from cyanosis, a blue coloring of the skin from lack of oxygen. The mottling is caused by an imbalance of the capillary squeezing motion, and it usually means patients are very close to death.

As people approach the time of death, their bodies let go of automated systems. And while the experience is unique for each dying patient, many share patterns and symptoms.

LOSING TOUCH WITH THE OUTSIDE WORLD

While a few people do remain conscious until the moment of death, this is the point when most dying people start to lose contact with the rest of the world if they haven't already. "I don't know if there's specifically, like a switch or something," says Hui. "We don't quite understand that—how do people who are still talking start to enter into those last days?"

In his book, *Palliative Care Perspectives*, Hallenbeck writes that patients seem to lose their senses and desires in a certain order. "First hunger and then thirst are lost," he writes.

This is, of course, different from patients who consciously choose to stop eating in order to hasten their deaths. Healthy people often worry that they or the people they love will experience suffering from starvation and thirst if they give up food and liquids as they die. That's not what the evidence indicates. Losing the desire to eat and drink is a natural part of the dying process, says Anne Rossignol, the Durango palliative care doctor. A study of patients with terminal cancer found that when they stopped eating, most did not experience hunger at all, and for the minority that did, the feeling disappeared quickly.

The sensations usually associated with dehydration—headaches, discomfort, thirst, nausea, cramps—are based on what healthy people feel, not what patients who are terminally ill experience. While dying people are often thirsty and say their mouths feel dry, this seems to be equally true both of patients who are dehydrated and those who are not. Family members and other caregivers will sometimes pressure patients to eat, but Rossignol tries to discourage this. At this point, food is "going to make [patients] feel bloated and give them diarrhea and nausea, and fluids are too; fluids are going to give them swelling and shortness of breath," she says. "So we're not helping them with those kinds of things." And providing nutrition artificially—through an IV tube, say—hasn't been shown to lengthen people's lives or reduce their suffering.

Sometimes, after dying patients stop eating, they will develop cravings for particular foods or drinks. "We had one guy who just loved his cup of coffee," Rossignol says. "And he couldn't swallow, he couldn't eat. The nurse . . . just got the tiniest little dropper and got him a little coffee, and he put it on his tongue and, 'Ohhhhhh,' and he closed his eyes, and he died."

After hunger and thirst disappear, speech is lost next, followed by vision. Even when patients are still conscious at this point, most are starting to lose touch with the outside world. According to one study, patients' ability to engage in complex communications fell to 15 percent in the twenty-four hours before dying.

"The last senses to go are usually hearing and touch," Hallenbeck concludes, echoing what many hospice and palliative care workers say.

How can researchers be sure those are the last senses to go? Neurologist James Bernat says this issue emphasizes the limitations of our knowledge about the dying experience. Patients usually have their eyes closed, so it's difficult to know whether they have the capacity to see, he points out. But their ears remain open, so it makes sense that hearing might be one of the last senses they experience.

It's important to remember that there are two components involved with any of our senses: One is the organ that does the sensing, and the second is the brain's processing of sensory input. When your eye is functioning normally, it sends signals to the occipital lobe cortex, where the brain interprets those signals as what you actually see. When you're dying, your eyes could be working fine, but your occipital lobe might be too damaged to translate signals into sight. The same is true for your ears. Sounds travel through the inner ear and are sent through the cranial nerve to the brain, and then on to the temporal lobe. Your sensory organs are more resistant than most brain cells are to the chemical breakdown that happens as you die. It's likely that your retina or your cochlea will work long after the relevant parts of the brain are able to process the information, because brain cells are more sensitive, Bernat says.

Bernat, like most doctors and nurses experienced in working with dying people, says he treats dying patients who appear unconscious as if they are conscious and capable of hearing. "We should be humble and assume that they are more able to hear us and understand some things than many people think they are," he says.

And sometimes, people who have been unconscious for days or weeks wake up just before they die.

TERMINAL LUCIDITY

This condition is common enough to have a name: terminal lucidity, "the so-called lucid interval that occurs during dying—where people will suddenly start talking in a very lucid way, as if somehow magically, they've regained certain functions that were assumed by family members were forever gone," says Bernat, who has witnessed these intervals. "It's very stunning to observe."

"It's the damndest thing," agrees Marian Grant, the hospice and palliative care nurse practitioner. "They are awake, they are present, they have sometimes very meaningful conversations with the people in their life, and then they die the next day. It's really mysterious."

Bernat has worked with some patients who have a combination of fatal brain hemorrhages and other severe conditions that have led family members to decide to stop providing treatments, he says. These patients usually stop receiving fluids, and they plunge into deep comas. Then, one or two days later, some patients suddenly open their eyes. Bernat theorizes that dehydration has reduced the brain's swelling, which in turn has reduced the brain pressure that led to the coma in the first place.

Grant has learned that this sudden return of lucidity doesn't indicate that a dying patient is improving. "It usually means that some big change is coming," she says. When it happens, she tells families, "'Please enjoy every minute of this, because this is probably not going to last, and this could be the beginning of the end as well.'" Sometimes, the condition lasts for minutes, sometimes an hour, but periods of terminal lucidity are transient. And then, ultimately, no one knows what people experience as their brains wind down. However, there is one area of clues: the firsthand accounts from people who have "near-death experiences."

NEAR-DEATH DESCRIPTIONS OFFER SOME HINTS ABOUT WHAT OUR FINAL EXPERIENCE MAY BE LIKE

In the stories about these experiences, the elements are now familiar: an out-of-body feeling; a journey through a dark tunnel; a bright light; a feeling of extreme clarity that makes the experiences seem more real than real life. Kevin Nelson, a neurology professor who has studied near-death experiences, says they don't provide scientific evidence of an afterlife. For one thing, the same experiences are described by people who are not close to death's door: Pilots in centrifuge often have out-of-body experiences, as do many people who faint.

But the experiences do provide crucial insights, Nelson believes: "I think the best glimpse we have for the dying brain are the people that don't die but come close." Many of the accounts of near-death experiences are reported by people who have survived cardiac arrest; while these people have not actually died, they have approached death as closely as anyone who is alive and able to talk about it has. And there is evidence that at least a small percentage of dying people will experience some of these phenomena.

It's important to remember that near-death phenomena are a rich set of experiences, and that there are multiple causes, Nelson says. "A lot of people are searching for *one* explanation. Well, it's actually a multitude of things that are going on."

As David Hovda, the UCLA Brain Injury Research Center director, explains, for example, one of the effects of the brain's deterioration can be seeing bright lights, another phenomenon reported in accounts of near-death experiences. This experience is connected to the way a healthy brain works: "Most of our mental activity is done through inhibition, not excitation," Hovda explains. That is, your brain spends a lot of its time and energy controlling urges and responses that are inappropriate. But when the brain starts to fail, it can no longer perform this job of inhibiting as well. "As the brain begins to change and starts to die, different parts become excited, and one of the parts that becomes excited is the visual system," Hovda says. "And so that's where people begin to see light."

That's how the brain's visual system knows how to respond, no matter what the stimulus: "If I put my finger in your eye— it's not going to be very pleasant for you—but what you're going to see when I do that is light, because the fibers in your retina respond to light," Hovda says. "So when they're activated, they tell the brain there's light out there, even though it's just my finger pushing on the eye."

Recent research points to evidence that the "more-real-than-real-life" experiences some people report also seem to match what we know about the brain's response to dying. Jimo Borjigin, the neuroscientist, said she hadn't been especially interested in studying death until she noticed something strange in the brains of animals in another experiment: Just before the animals died, neurochemicals in the brain suddenly surged. While scientists had known that brain neurons continued to fire after a person died, this was different. The neurons were secreting new chemicals, and in large amounts.

Borjigin delved into the literature about near-death experiences. "I realized, a lot of cardiac arrest survivors describe that during their unconscious period, they have this amazing experience in their brain," she says. "They see lights and then they describe the experience as 'realer than real.'" And she realized the sudden release of neurochemicals might help to explain the "realer than real" feeling.

Borjigin and her research team tried an experiment: They anesthetized eight rats, and then stopped their hearts.

"Suddenly, all the different regions of the brain became synchronized—they were firing in synchrony," she said. After further analysis, the researchers measured one particular frequency, the gamma frequency, and found that it was above 25 hertz. "And that's really intense," she says. The brain was "super-alert, very much alerted to the absent supply of oxygen."

The rats' brains showed both higher power in different frequency waves, and also coherence, or the electrical activity from different parts of the brain working together.

"If you're focusing attention, doing something, trying to figure out a word or trying to remember a face—when you're doing high-level cognitive activity, these features go up," Borjigin says. "These are well-used parameters in studying human consciousness in awake humans. So, we thought, if you're alert or aroused, similar parameters should also go up in the dying brain. In fact, that was the case."

And the results matched the near-death reports of experiences growing sharper: "If I have neurochemical secretions suddenly surge ten- to twenty-fold higher than the daytime level, when I'm awake, I might think that's realer than real."

But near-death experiences are individual, internal experiences, she notes. "You cannot reproduce somebody else's near-death experience, even if you go through exactly the same dying experience."

THE LAST MINUTES

Just as my mother's hospice nurse did, Hallenbeck sometimes asks patients if they'd like to know what they'll probably experience as they die. Most do, he says, although they're often nervous about what he'll have to say.

He tells them, "What usually happens is, people get tired and weak, and kind of go off to sleep. It's kind of like going to sleep, the best I can tell." Falling asleep is different for different people—some people have worse insomnia, and some people just drop off immediately, and he believes dying is similar in that sense. But the experience doesn't seem terrible, he says.

In patients' final hours, after they've stopped eating and drinking, after they've lost their vision, "Most dying people then close their eyes and appear to be asleep. From this point on, dying is very mysterious, and we can only infer what is actually happening," Hallenbeck says. "My impression is that this is not a coma, a state of unconsciousness, as many families and clinicians think, but something like a dream state."

"I've often compared dying to black holes: We can see the effect of black holes, but it is extremely difficult, if not impossible, to look inside them," Hallenbeck wrote to me. "They exert an increasingly strong gravitational pull the closer one gets to them. As one passes the 'event horizon,' apparently the laws of physics begin to change." Researchers and doctors can examine dying patients' symptoms and behaviors and estimate or guess what they're feeling physically or, sometimes, even consciously. But as patients approach closer and closer to death, it's harder and harder for doctors to know for certain what they're experiencing.

Campbell puts it like this: "It's like a big, dark hole of we-don't-know-what's-going-on in that period."

A black hole. A black box. A dark hole.

What that final, physical experience of dying—the last few days or moments—is like may never be fully understood. The exact moment when we enter a dream state, or even when we start dying, is hard to pinpoint. "It's like a storm coming in," Hallenbeck says. "The waves started coming up. But you can never say, well, when did the waves start coming up? I don't know. Is it a ripple? Is it this big? Is it two feet?

"The waves get higher and higher and, eventually, they carry the person out to sea."

CODA

I don't remember the exact words that Pat Amthor, the hospice nurse, used when she told my mother and me what would happen as she died. So I asked Pat—and Michelle Appenzeller, and Marian Grant, and Anne Rossignol, and Deb Callahan— What do you say to dying patients, especially those with advanced breast cancer, who want to know what those final days feel like?

The following is a compilation of what they told me.

Everyone's death is different. I compare it to the birth stories that women always give. With dying, it's the same thing: It's different for everyone. There's no textbook. And the guidelines are just that—they're guidelines.

When your body starts to shut down, your organs also begin breaking down: Your lungs stop working as well, your heart doesn't beat as well, your kidneys don't remove toxins as efficiently. And the gradual loss of any organ affects your whole system. If your kidneys aren't working, toxins build up and affect your brain. If your heart isn't pumping well, your brain isn't getting enough oxygen. If your brain isn't functioning properly, it's not telling the rest of the body what to do. As nurses or doctors, we observe, "Gosh, your feet are mottling. You're not having perfusion to your feet—you don't have good circulation." Your hands don't pink up so well; they get to be gray. You become more ashen.

You will lose your appetite, and you'll give up eating and drinking—that's a very natural part of the dying process. Then you're looking at days. Bodies need hydration, so then the kidneys start to fail, which is actually very anesthetic. Bodies know how to die. We try to encourage families, because people love with food in this country, not to pressure patients to eat. At some point, food is going to make you feel bloated and give you diarrhea and nausea, and fluids are, too; fluids are going to give you swelling and shortness of breath. Let it happen, and we will treat the symptoms.

You will likely become fatigued and then very sleepy, and your desire to interact with people will dwindle. You'll be less interested in visitors, and less interactive with your family. Even your surroundings—who's coming in the door, what's going on outside your window—will probably hold less interest for you. Your brain is shutting down.

This is a normal, natural process that happens, but I don't think it's always that comfortable for people. When I'm caring for a patient, I reassure them that I'm going to be able to manage all those symptoms, and we can anticipate them. That's our job, and that's why we have hospice: to be able to anticipate and prevent, or minimize, suffering. Sometimes, you will have increased pain, which is evidence of the spreading of disease. You might have other symptoms: difficulty breathing, that kind of thing. It can feel like you can't get enough air—that's the dyspnea, or air hunger—that's a very uncomfortable feeling, but it can also be treated.

If you have heart disease, sometimes people begin having trouble with swallowing because the heart can't pump as much. You can't take diuretics to make you pee as much, so you might get some swelling; that's when the lungs start to fill up, because you can't manage all those secretions. And that's when we give you medications to dry things out, and then there's a whole thing where the throat starts to relax so much and there's this gurgling that happens. You aren't all that uncomfortable, but the people observing that are very uncomfortable.

*As your organs continue to break down, you'll
probably sink into unconsciousness more and more.
That's a normal process. What can happen is you are
really starting to get that sense of what's next. You might
experience terminal agitation, where you're trying to
get up out of bed, swatting at things, and, depending
on your age, pacing around the floor; you just can't get
comfortable. It's like you're out of your skin. What we try
to do when we give medication is to help you feel relaxed
around it. You can get comfortable with that process
that's happening, because it's natural. It is a natural
process.*

*Pain seems to dissipate in the very last few hours,
and, for most people, those hours are peaceful.*

Bodies know how to die.—PAT AMTHOR, FORMER
DURANGO HOSPICE NURSE; MICHELLE APPENZELLER,
CLINICAL DIRECTOR AT HOSPICE OF MERCY IN DURANGO;
ANNE ROSSIGNOL, DURANGO PALLIATIVE CARE DOCTOR; DEB
CALLAHAN, HOSPICE VOLUNTEER AND FORMER HOSPICE NURSE;
MARIAN GRANT, HOSPICE AND PALLIATIVE CARE NURSE
PRACTITIONER AND SENIOR ADVISER TO THE COALITION TO
TRANSFORM ADVANCED CARE

bibliography

Alici, Y., & Breitbart, W. (2009, May). Delirium in palliative care. *Primary Psychiatry, 16*(5): 42–48.

Aragon, K., Covinsky, K., Miao, Y., Boscardin, W.J., Flint, L., & Smith, A.K. (2012, November 12). Use of the Medicare posthospitalization skilled nursing benefit in the last 6 months of life. *Archives of Internal Medicine, 172*(20): 1573–1579.

Barskova, T., & Oesterreich, R. (2009). Post-traumatic growth in people living with a serious medical condition and its relations to physical and mental health: A systematic review. *Disability and Rehabilitation, 31*(21): 1709–1733.

Baxter, A. (2017, October 8). What hospice care looks like in America. *Home Health Care News.* Retrieved March 6, 2018, from homehealthcarenews.com/2017/10/what-hospice -care-looks-like-in-america.

Bekelman, J., Halpern, S.D., Blankart, C.R., Bynum, J.P., Cohen, J., Fowler, R., . . . & Emanuel, E.J. (2016, January 19). Comparison of site of death, health care utilization, and hospital expenditures for patients dying with cancer in 7 developed countries. *Journal of the American Medical Association, 315*(3): 272–283.

Blinderman, C. D., & Cherny, N. I. (2005). Existential issues do not necessarily result in existential suffering: Lessons from cancer patients in Israel. *Palliative Medicine, 19*: 371–380.

Boly, M., Faymonville, M.E., Schnakers, C., Peigneux, P., Lambermont, B., Phillips, C., . . . & Laureys, S. (2008, November). Perception of pain in the minimally conscious state with PET activation: An observational study. *The Lancet Neurology (11)*: 1013–1020.

Breitbart, W., Gibson, C., & Tremblay, A. (2002, May–June). The delirium experience: Delirium recall and delirium-related distress in hospitalized patients with cancer, their spouses/caregivers, and their nurses. *Psychosomatics 43*(3): 183–194.

Byock, I. (1995, March/April). Patient refusal of nutrition and hydration: Walking the ever-finer line. *American Journal of Hospice & Palliative Care:* 8–13.

———. (1996). The nature of suffering and the nature of opportunity at the end of life. *Clinics in Geriatric Medicine, 12*(2): 237–252.

———. (1997). *Dying well: Peace and possibilities at the end of life.* New York: Riverhead Books.

———. (2004, 2014). *The four things that matter most: A book about living.* New York: Atria Books.

———. (2008). Personal growth and human development in life-threatening conditions: Therapeutic insights and strategies derived from positive experiences of individuals and families. In H. Chochinov & W. Breitbart (Eds.), *Handbook of Psychiatry in Palliative Medicine* (pp. 281–299). Oxford: Oxford University Press.

Calhoun, L.G., & Tedeschi, R.G. (2004). The foundations of posttraumatic growth: New considerations. *Psychological Inquiry, 15*(1): 93–102.

———. (2013). *Posttraumatic growth in clinical practice.* New York: Routledge.

Campbell, M.L., & Yarandi, H.N. (2013). Death rattle is not associated with patient respiratory distress: Is pharmacologic treatment indicated? *Journal of Palliative Medicine, 16*(10): 1255–1259.

Cassell, E.J. (1982, March 18). The nature of suffering and the goals of medicine. *The New England Journal of Medicine, 306*(11): 639–645.

———. (1991, 2004). *The nature of suffering and the goals of medicine.* New York: Oxford University Press.

Centers for Disease Control and Prevention. National Center for Health Statistics. Underlying cause of death 1999–2016 on CDC WONDER Online Database, released December 2017.

Christakis, N.A., & Lamont, E.B. (2000, February 19). Extent and determinants of error in doctors' prognoses in terminally ill patients: A prospective cohort study. *The BMJ, 320*(7233): 469–473.

Clark, D. (Ed.). (2002). *Cicely Saunders: Founder of the Hospice Movement, Selected Letters 1959-1999.* New York: Oxford University Press.

———. (2006). *Cicely Saunders: Selected writings 1958-2004.* Oxford, UK: Oxford University Press.

Clemons, M., Regnard, C., & Appleton, T. (1996). Alertness, cognition and morphine in patients with advanced cancer. *Cancer Treatment Reviews, 22*: 451–468.

Coleman, M.R., Rodd, J.M., Davis, M.H., Johnsrude, I.S., Menon, D.K., Pickard, J.D., & Owen, A.M. (2007). Do vegetative patients retain aspects of language comprehension? Evidence from fMRI. *Brain, 130*: 2494–2507.

Coyle, N. (2004). The existential slap—A crisis of disclosure. *International Journal of Palliative Nursing, 10*(11): 520.

———. (2004, April). In their own words: Seven advanced cancer patients describe their experience with pain and the use of opioid drugs. *Journal of pain and symptom management, 27*(4): 300–309.

———. (2006, September). The hard work of living in the face of death. *Journal of Pain and Symptom Management, 32*(3): 266–274.

De Graeff, A., & Dean, M. (2007). Palliative sedation therapy in the last weeks of life: A literature review and recommendations for standards. *Journal of Palliative Medicine, 10*(1): 67–85.

Eddy, D. (1994, July 20). A conversation with my mother. *Journal of the American Medical Association, 272*(3): 179–181.

Ellershaw, J.E., Sutcliffe, J.M., & Saunders, C.M. (1995, April). Dehydration and the dying patient. *Journal of Pain and Symptom Management, 10*(3): 192–197.

Emanuel, E.J., Onwuteaka-Philpsen, B.D., Urwin, J.W., & Cohen, J. (2016). Attitudes and practices of euthanasia and physician-assisted suicide in the United States, Canada, and Europe. *Journal of the American Medical Association, 316*(1): 79–90.

Erikson, E.H. (1950, 1993). *Childhood and society.* New York: W.W. Norton.

Ferris, F, von Gunten, C., & Emanuel, L. (2003, August). Competency in end-of-life care: Last hours of life. *Journal of Palliative Medicine, 6*(4): 605–613.

Fine, R.L. (2007, January). Ethical and practical issues with opioids in life-limiting illness. *Proceedings of Baylor University Medical Center, 20*(1): 5–12.

Flemming, K. (2010, January). The use of morphine to treat cancer-related pain: A synthesis of quantitative and qualitative research. *Journal of Pain and Symptom Management, 39*(1): 139–154.

Flory, J., Young-Xu, Y., Gurol, I., Levinsky, N., Ash, A., &

Emanuel, E. (2004, May). Place of death: U.S. trends since 1980. *Health Affairs, 23*(3): 194–200.

García-Rueda, N. Valcárcel, A.C., Saracíbar-Razquin, M.S., & Solabarrieta, M.A. (2016, April). The experience of living with advanced-stage cancer: A thematic synthesis of the literature. *European Journal of Cancer Care, 25*: 551–569. doi: 10.1111/ecc.12523

Gawande, A. (2008, June 30). The itch: Its mysterious power may be a clue to a new theory about brains and bodies. *The New Yorker.* Retrieved September 8, 2017, from www.newyorker.com/magazine/2008/06/30/the-itch.

Glare, P., Virik, K., Jones, M., Hudson, M., Eychmuller, S., Simes, J., & Christakis, N. (2003, July 26). A systematic review of physicians' survival predictions in terminally ill cancer patients. *The BMJ, 327*(7408): 195–198.

Glaser, B.G., & Strauss, A.L. (1968). *Time for dying* (2nd ed.). Chicago: Aldine Publishing.

Hallenbeck, J. (2003). *Palliative Care Perspectives.* New York: Oxford University Press.

———. (2008, June/July). Access to end-of-life care venues. *American Journal of Hospice & Palliative Medicine, 25*(3): 245–249.

Howell, D., Fitch, M.I., & Deane, K.A. (2003). Impact of ovarian cancer perceived by women. *Cancer Nursing, 26*(1): 1–9.

IASP Terminology. (2017, December 14). In International Association for the Study of Pain. Retrieved April 29, 2018, from www.iasp-pain.org/Education/Content.aspx?ItemNumber=1698.

Jones, D.S., Podolsky, S.H., & Greene, J.A. (2012, June 21). The burden of disease and the changing task of medicine. *New England Journal of Medicine, 366.* doi: 10.1056/NEJMp1113569

Kamal, A., Taylor, D.H., Neely, B., Harker, M., Bhullar, P., Morris, J., . . . & Bull, J. (2017, October). One size does not fit all: Disease profiles of serious illness patients receiving specialty palliative care. *Journal of Pain and Symptom Management, 54*(4): 476–483.

Kendall, M., Carduff, E., Lloyd, A., Kimbell, B., Cavers, D., Buckingham, S., . . . & Murray, S.A. (2015, August). Different experiences and goals in different advanced diseases: Comparing serial interviews with patients with cancer, organ failure, or frailty and their family and professional careers. *Journal of Pain and Symptom Management, 50*(2): 216–224.

Kerr, C.W., Donnelly, J.P., Wright, S.T., Kuszczak, S.M., Banas, A., Grant, P.C., & Luczkiewicz, D.L. (2014). End-of-life dreams and visions: A longitudinal study of hospice patients' experiences. *Journal of Palliative Medicine, 17*(3): 296–303.

Kochanek, K.D., Murphy, S.L., Xu, J., & Arias, E. (2017, December). Mortality in the United States, 2016. *NCHS Data Brief, 293*: 1–8.

Kübler-Ross, E. (1969, 2003). *On death and dying: What the dying have to teach doctors, nurses, clergy and their own families.* New York: Scribner.

Kushner, H.S. (1981). *When bad things happen to good people.* New York: Anchor Books.

Kwoh, C.K., O'Connor, G.T., Regan-Smith, M.G., Olmstead, E.M., Brown, L.A., Burnett, J.B., . . . & Morgan, G.J. (1992). Concordance between clinician and patient assessment of physical and mental health status. *The Journal of Rheumatology, 19*(7): 1031–1037.

Lederle, F. (2017, December 5). Terminal. *Annals of Internal Medicine, 167*(11): 826–827.

Lee, V. (2008). The existential plight of cancer: Meaning

making as a concrete approach to the intangible search for meaning. *Support Care Cancer, 16*: 779–785.

Levenson, J.W., McCarthy, E.P., Lynn J., Davis R.B., & Phillips, R.S. (2000, May). The last six months of life for patients with congestive heart failure. *Journal of the American Geriatrics Society, 48*(5 Suppl): S101-9.

Leveton, A. (1965). Time, death and the ego-chill. *Journal of Existentialism, 6*(21): 69–80.

Lichter, I., & Hunt, E. (1990). The last 48 hours of life. *Journal of Palliative Care, 6*(4): 7–15.

Lunney, J.R., Lynn, J., Foley, D.J., Lipson, S., & Guralnik, J.M. (2003, May 14). Patterns of functional decline at the end of life. *Journal of the American Medical Association, 289*(18): 2387–2392.

Lunney, J.R., Lynn, J., & Hogan, C. (2002). Profiles of older Medicare decedents. *Journal of the American Geriatrics Society, 50:* 1108–1112.

Lynn, J. (2005). Living long in fragile health: The new demographics shape end of life care. *Hastings Center Report*, Nov.–Dec. Spec. No. S14-18.

———. (2008, April 24). Reliable comfort and meaningfulness. *The BMJ, 336*: 958.

———. (2017, Oct. 18). Traveling the valley of the shadow of death in 2017. *Health Affairs Blog, 36*(10): 1695–1854.

Mann, T. (1996, 1924). *The Magic Mountain*. New York: Vintage Books.

McCann, R.M., Hall, W.J., & Groth-Juncker, A.G. (1994, October 26). Comfort care for terminally ill patients: The appropriate use of nutrition and hydration. *Journal of the American Medical Association, 272*(16): 1263–1266.

Meldrum, M.L. (2003, November 12). A capsule history of pain management. *Journal of the American Medical Association, 290*(18): 2470–2475.

Missel, M., & Birkelund, R. (2011). Living with incurable oesophageal cancer: A phenomenological hermeneutical interpretation of patient stories. *European Journal of Oncology Nursing, 15*: 296–301.

Monti, M.M., Vanhaudenhuyse, A., Coleman, M.R., Boly, M., Pickard, J.D., Tshibanda, L., . . . & Laureys, S. (2010, February 10). Willful modulation of brain activity in disorders of consciousness. *New England Journal of Medicine, 362*(7): 579–589.

Morita, T., Ichiki, T., Tsunoda, J., Inoue, S., & Chihara, S. (1998, July/August). A prospective study on the dying process in terminally ill cancer patients. *The American Journal of Hospice & Palliative Care, 15*(4): 217–222.

Morita, T., Tei, Y., & Inoue, S. (2003, September). Impaired communication capacity and agitated delirium in the final week of terminally ill cancer patients: Prevalence and identification of research focus. *Journal of Pain and Symptom Management, 26*(3): 827–834.

Mount, B.M., Boston, P.H., & Cohen, S.R. (2007, April). Healing connections: On moving from suffering to a sense of well-being. *Journal of Pain and Symptom Management, 33*(4): 372–388.

Murray, K. (2011, November 30). How doctors die. *Zócalo Public Square.* Retrieved August 10, 2017, from www .zocalopublicsquare.org/2011/11/30/how-doctors-die/ideas /nexus.

Mystakidou, K., Tsilika, E., Parpa, E., Kyriakopoulos, D., Malamos, N., & Damigos, D. (2008). Personal growth and psychological distress in advanced breast cancer. *The Breast, 17*: 382–386.

Naro, A., Leo, A., Cannavò A., Buda, A., Bramanti, P., & Calabrò R.S. (2016, March). Do unresponsive wakefulness syndrome patients feel pain? Role of laser-evoked potential-induced gamma-band oscillations in detecting cortical pain processing. *Neuroscience, 317*: 141–148.

National Hospice and Palliative Care Organization. (2018, March). NHPCO facts and figures: Hospice care in America. Alexandria, VA. Retrieved February 8, 2017, from www.nhpco.org/sites/default/files/public/Statistics_Research/2017_Facts_Figures.pdf.

National Institute on Drug Abuse. (2018, March). Opioid overdose crisis. Retrieved May 10, 2018, from www.drugabuse.gov/drugs-abuse/opioids/opioid-overdose-crisis#one.

Nissim, R., Freeman, E., Lo, C., Zimmermann, C., Gagliese, L., Rydall, A., . . . & Rodin, G. (2011). Managing cancer and living meaningfully (CALM): A qualitative study of a brief individual psychotherapy for individuals with advanced cancer. *Palliative Medicine, 26*(5): 713–721.

Nissim, R., Rennie, D., Fleming, S., Hales, S., Gagliese, L., & Rodin, G. (2012). Goals set in the land of the living/dying: A longitudinal study of patients living with advanced cancer. *Death Studies, 36*: 360–390.

Nuland, S.B. (1993/1995). *How we die: Reflections on life's final chapter.* New York: Vintage Books.

Oregon Public Health Division, Center for Health Statistics. (2018, February 9). Oregon Death with Dignity Act: Data Summary 2017. p. 5. Retrieved May 17, 2018, from www.oregon.gov.

Owen, A. (2017). *Into the gray zone: A neuroscientist explores the border between life and death.* New York: Scribner.

Pattison, E.M. (1977). *The experience of dying.* Englewood Cliffs, NJ: Prentice Hall.

Perrin, F., Schnakers, C., Schabus, M., Degueldre, C., Goldman, S., Brédart, S., . . . & Laureys, S. (2006, April). Brain response to one's own name in vegetative state, minimally conscious state, and locked-in syndrome. *Archives of Neurology, 63*: 562–569.

Plonk, W.M., & Armold, R.M. (2005). Terminal care: The last weeks of life. *Journal of Palliative Medicine, 8*(5): 1042–1054.

Pollock, K. (2015, October). Is home always the best and preferred place of death? *The BMJ, 7*(351): 1–3.

Pritchard, R.S., Fisher, E., Teno, J.M., & Lynn, J. (1998, October). Influence of patient preferences and local health system characteristics on the place of death. *Journal of the American Geriatrics Society, 46*(10): 1242–1250.

Rabkin, J.G., Albert, S.M., Del Bene, M.L., O'Sullivan, I., Tider, T., Rowland, L.P., & Mitsumoto, H. (2005, September 13). Prevalence of depressive disorders and change over time in late-stage ALS. *Neurology, 65*(1): 62–67.

Remington, R., & Wakim, G. (2010, August 23). A comparison of hospice in the United States and the United Kingdom. *Journal of Gerontological Nursing, 36*(9): 16–21.

Romem, A., Tom, S.E., Beauchene, M., Babington, L., & Scharf, S.M. (2015). Pain management at the end of life: A comparative study of cancer, dementia, and chronic obstructive pulmonary disease patients. *Palliative Medicine, 29*(5): 464–469.

Sacks, O. (2015, February 19). My own life. *New York Times.* Retrieved July 6, 2017, from www.nytimes.com.

Schulz, U., & Mohamed, N.E. (2004). Turning the tide: Benefit finding after cancer. *Social Science & Medicine, 59*: 653–662.

Schwarz, J. (2011). Death by voluntary dehydration: Suicide or the right to refuse a life-prolonging measure? *Widener Law Review, 17*(351): 351–361.

Singer, A.E., Meeker, D., Teno, J.M., Lynn, J., Lunney, J.R., & Lorenz, K.A. (2015). Symptom trends in the last year of life from 1998 to 2010: A cohort study. *Annals of Internal Medicine, 162*(3): 175–188.

Solano, J.P., Gomes, B., & Higginson, I.J. (2006, January). A comparison of symptom prevalence in far advanced cancer, AIDS, heart disease, chronic obstructive pulmonary disease and renal disease. *Journal of Pain and Symptom Management, 31*(1): 58–69.

Srivastava, R. (2017, May 1). Dying at home might sound preferable. But I've seen the reality. *The Guardian.*

Steinfels, P. (1996, November 15). Cardinal Bernardin dies at 68; Reconciling voice in church. *New York Times.*

Steinhauser, K.E., Arnold, R.M., Olsen, M.K., Lindquist, J., Hays, J., Wood, L.L., . . . & Tulsky, J.A. (2011, September). Comparing three life-limiting diseases: Does diagnosis matter or is sick, sick? *Journal of Pain and Symptom Management, 42*(3): 331–341.

Sullivan, A.D., Hedberg, K., & Fleming, D.W. (2000, February 24). Legalized physician-assisted suicide in Oregon—The second year. *New England Journal of Medicine, 342*: 598–604.

Tang, S.T. (2003). When death is imminent: Where terminally ill patients with cancer prefer to die and why. *Cancer Nursing, 26*(3): 245–251.

Tang, S.T., Lin, K.C., Chen, J.S., Chang, W.C., Hsieh, C.H., & Chou, W.C. (2015). Threatened with death but growing: Changes in and determinants of posttraumatic growth over the dying process for Taiwanese terminally ill cancer patients. *Psycho-Oncology, 24*: 147–154.

Taylor, E.J. (2000). Transformation of tragedy among women surviving breast cancer. *Oncology Nursing Forum, 27*(5): 781–788.

Tedeschi, R., & Calhoun, L. (2004). Posttraumatic growth: Conceptual foundations and empirical evidence. *Psychological Inquiry, 15*(1): 1–18.

Tempelaar, R., De Haes, J.C., De Ruiter, J.H., Bakker, D., Van Den Heuvel, W.J., & Van Nieuwenhuijzen, M.G. (1989). The social experiences of cancer under treatment: A comparative study. *Social Science Medicine, 29*(5): 635–642.

Teno, J.M., Clarridge, B.R., Casey, V., Welch, L.C., Wetle, T., Shield, R., & Mor, V. (2004, January 7). Family perspectives on end-of-life care at the last place of care. *Journal of the American Medical Association, 291*(1): 88–93.

Teno, J.M., Freedman, V.A., Kasper, J.D., Gozalo, P. & Mor, V. (2015). Is care for the dying improving in the United States? *Journal of Palliative Medicine, 1*(8): 662–666.

Teno, J.M., Gozalo, P.L., Bynum, J.P.W., Leland, N.E., Miller, S.C., Morden, N.E., . . . & Mor, V. (2013, February 6). Change in end-of-life care for Medicare beneficiaries: Site of death, place of care, and health care transitions in 2000, 2005, and 2009. *Journal of the American Medical Association, 309*(5): 470–477.

Teno, J.M., Weitzen, S., Fennell, M.L., & Mor, V. (2001). Dying trajectory in the last year of life: Does cancer trajectory fit other diseases? *Journal of Palliative Medicine, 4*(4): 457–464.

Thomas, C., Morris, S.M., & Clark, D. (2004). Place of death: Preferences among cancer patients and their carers. *Social Science & Medicine, 58*: 2431–2444.

Weisman, A. (1972). *On dying and denying.* New York: Behavioral Publications.

Weisman, A., & Worden, J.W. (1976). The existential plight in cancer: Significance of the first 100 days. *International Journal of Psychiatry in Medicine, 7*(1): 1–15.

Weiss, S.C., Emanuel, L.L., Fairclough, D.L., & Emanuel, E.J. (2001, April 28). Understanding the experience of pain in terminally ill patients. *The Lancet, 357*: 1311–1314.

Widows, M.R., Jacobsen, P.B., Booth-Jones, M., & Fields, K.K. (2005). Predictors of posttraumatic growth following bone marrow transplantation for cancer. *Health Psychology, 24*(3): 266–273.

Winter, S.M. (2000, December 15). Terminal nutrition: Framing the debate for the withdrawal of nutritional support in terminally ill patients. *The American Journal of Medicine, 109*: 723–726.

Wrubel, J., Acree, M., Goodman S., & Folkman, S. (2009, December). End of living: Maintaining a lifeworld during terminal illness. *Psychology and Health, 24*(10): 1229–1243.

notes

INTRODUCTION

4: more than 90 percent of all Americans Ferris, F., von Gunten, C., & Emanuel, L. (2003, August). Competency in end-of-life care: Last hours of life. *Journal of Palliative Medicine, 6*(4): 605–613, p. 605.

CHAPTER ONE: EXISTENTIAL SLAP: A FATAL DIAGNOSIS

9: this awareness precipitates a crisis for most individuals Coyle, N. (2004). The existential slap—a crisis of disclosure. *International Journal of Palliative Nursing, 10*(11): 520.

10: people are used to being vulnerable Missel, M., & Birkelund, R. (2011). Living with incurable oesophageal cancer: A phenomenological hermeneutical interpretation of patient stories. *European Journal of Oncology Nursing, 15:* 296–301, p. 296.

we anticipate a certain life-span Pattison, E.M. (1977). *The experience of dying* (p. 44). Englewood Cliffs, NJ: Prentice Hall.

good people deserve good things happening to them Lee, V. (2008). The existential plight of cancer: Meaning making as a concrete approach to the intangible search for meaning. *Support Care Cancer, 16*: 779–785.

11: I couldn't handle the future Missel, M., & Birkelund, R. (2011). Living with incurable oesophageal cancer: A phenomenological hermeneutical interpretation of patient stories. *European Journal of Oncology Nursing, 15:* 296–301, p. 298.

almost every aspect of life Lee, V. (2008). The existential plight of cancer: Meaning making as a concrete approach to the intangible search for meaning. *Support Care Cancer, 16*: 779–785, p. 785.

Avery Weisman and J. William Worden Weisman, A., & Worden, J.W. (1976). The existential plight in cancer: Significance of the first 100 days. *International Journal of Psychiatry in Medicine, 7*(1): 1–15.

15: middle knowledge Weisman, A. (1972). *On dying and denying.* New York: Behavioral Publications.

CHAPTER TWO: TRAJECTORIES: PATTERNS IN HOW WE DIE

20: a fourth graph described by Joanne Lynn Lunney, J.R., Lynn, J., & Hogan, C. (2002). Profiles of older Medicare decedents. *Journal of the American Geriatrics Society, 50*: 1108–1112; Lunney, J.R., Lynn, J., Foley, D.J., Lipson, S., & Guralnik, J.M. (2003, May 14). Patterns of functional decline at the end of life. *Journal of the American Medical Association, 289*(18): 2387–2392.

until his last days Steinfels, P. (1996, November 15). Cardinal Bernardin dies at 68: Reconciling voice in church. *New York Times.*

21: the way we imagine death and the way it's more likely to transpire Glaser, B.G., & Strauss, A.L. (1968). *Time for dying* (2nd ed.). Chicago: Aldine Publishing.

27: the majority of hospice patients in the United States

had cancer Kamal, A., Taylor, D.H., Neely, B., Harker, M., Bhullar, P., Morris, J., . . . & Bull, J. (2017, October). One size does not fit all: Disease profiles of serious illness patients receiving specialty palliative care. *Journal of Pain and Symptom Management, 54*(4): 476–483, p. 477.

30: live with a fatal condition Kendall, M., Carduff, E., Lloyd, A., Kimbell, B., Cavers, D., Buckingham, S., . . . & Murray, S.A. (2015, August). Different experiences and goals in different advanced diseases: Comparing serial interviews with patients with cancer, organ failure, or frailty and their family and professional careers. *Journal of Pain and Symptom Management, 50*(2): 216–224.

31: while this increase in longevity Solano, J.P., Gomes, B., & Higginson, I.J. (2006, January). A comparison of symptom prevalence in far advanced cancer, AIDS, heart disease, chronic obstructive pulmonary disease and renal disease. *Journal of Pain and Symptom Management, 31*(1): 58–69, pp. 58, 64.

losing nearly half of her weight Lynn, J. (2017, October 18). Traveling the valley of the shadow of death in 2017. *Health Affairs Blog, 36*(10): 1695–1854.

34: ten most common causes of death in the United States Kochanek, K.D., Murphy, S.L., Xu, J., & Arias, E. (2017, December). Mortality in the United States, 2016. *NCHS Data Brief, 293*: 1–8.

35: to prevent one way of dying Hallenbeck, J. (2003). *Palliative care perspectives* (p. 2). New York: Oxford University Press.

36: compared cancer patients' symptoms Solano, J.P., Gomes, B., & Higginson, I.J. (2006, January). A comparison of symptom prevalence in far advanced cancer, AIDS, heart disease, chronic obstructive pulmonary disease and renal disease. *Journal of Pain and Symptom Management, 31*(1): 58–69.

a common pathway Solano, J.P., Gomes, B., & Higginson,

I.J. (2006, January). A comparison of symptom prevalence in far advanced cancer, AIDS, heart disease, chronic obstructive pulmonary disease and renal disease. *Journal of Pain and Symptom Management, 31*(1): 58–69, p. 64.

36: does diagnosis matter or is sick, sick Steinhauser, K.E., Arnold, R.M., Olsen, M.K., Lindquist, J., Hays, J., Wood, L.L., . . . & Tulsky, J.A. (2011, September). Comparing three life-limiting diseases: Does diagnosis matter or is sick, sick? *Journal of Pain and Symptom Management, 42*(3): 331–341.

significant effects on patients' quality of life Steinhauser, K.E., Arnold, R.M., Olsen, M.K., Lindquist, J., Hays, J., Wood, L.L., . . . & Tulsky, J.A. (2011, September). Comparing three life-limiting diseases: Does diagnosis matter or is sick, sick? *Journal of Pain and Symptom Management, 42*(3): 331–341, p. 335.

37: ability to participate in daily activities Teno, J.M., Weitzen, S., Fennell, M.L., & Mor, V. (2001). Dying trajectory in the last year of life: Does cancer trajectory fit other diseases? *Journal of Palliative Medicine, 4*(4): 457–464.

50 percent of non-cancer patients shared this difficulty Teno, J.M., Weitzen, S., Fennell, M.L., & Mor, V. (2001). Dying trajectory in the last year of life: Does cancer trajectory fit other diseases? *Journal of Palliative Medicine, 4*(4): 457–464, p. 457.

CHAPTER THREE: AFTER THE DIAGNOSIS: IN THE LAND OF LIVING/DYING

40: an unnatural place in which to live Nissim, R., Rennie, D., Fleming, S., Hales, S., Gagliese, L., & Rodin, G. (2012). Goals set in the land of the living/dying: A longitudinal study of patients living with advanced cancer. *Death Studies, 36*: 360–390, p. 368.

the continual knowing Nissim, R., Rennie, D., Fleming, S., Hales, S., Gagliese, L., & Rodin, G. (2012). Goals set in the land of the living/dying: A longitudinal study of patients living with advanced cancer. *Death Studies, 36*: 360–390, pp. 368–369.

he's not dying yet Lynn, J. (2005). Living long in fragile health: The new demographics shape end of life care. *Hastings Center Report*, Nov.-Dec. Spec. No. S14-18, p. S14.

41: we are not half dead people who cannot do anything Mount, B.M., Boston, P.H., & Cohen, S.R. (2007, April). Healing connections: On moving from suffering to a sense of well-being. *Journal of Pain and Symptom Management, 33*(4): 372–388, p. 377.

Elisabeth Kübler-Ross's five stages of grief Kübler-Ross, E. (1969, 2003). *On death and dying: What the dying have to teach doctors, nurses, clergy and their own families.* New York: Scribner.

the dying were moved out of homes and into hospitals This move, by the way, seems to have been the result of several factors: Hospitals had begun to transform from glorified almshouses into more respectable institutions, and the public became more aware of that trend as soldiers were treated at hospitals during the Civil War. At the same time, more Americans were moving farther away from their families, and more advanced medical technology was becoming available in hospitals that wasn't available in private homes.

42: *I did not go through the five stages* Lederle, F. (2017, December 5) Terminal. *Annals of Internal Medicine*, 167(11): 826–827

43: the leading causes of death at the time Jones, D.S., Podolsky, S.H., & Greene, J.A. (2012, June 21). The burden of disease and the changing task of medicine. *New England Journal of Medicine, 366*. doi: 10.1056/NEJMp1113569

46: a group of Spanish nurses García-Rueda, N., Valcárcel, A.C., Saracíbar-Razquin, M.S., & Solabarrieta, M.A. (2016, April). The experience of living with advanced-stage cancer:

A thematic synthesis of the literature. *European Journal of Cancer Care, 25*: 551–569.

47: seriously ill people may rate life quality even more highly Mount, B.M., Boston, P.H., & Cohen, S.R. (2007, April). Healing connections: On moving from suffering to a sense of well-being. *Journal of Pain and Symptom Management, 33*(4): 372–388, p. 373.

few of the patients were depressed Rabkin, J.G., Albert, S.M., Del Bene, M.L., O'Sullivan, I., Tider, T., Rowland, L.P., & Mitsumoto, H. (2005, September 13). Prevalence of depressive disorders and change over time in late-stage ALS. *Neurology, 65*(1): 62–67.

perceived quality of life didn't decline significantly Levenson, J.W., McCarthy, E.P., Lynn J., Davis R.B., & Phillips, R.S. (2000, May). The last six months of life for patients with congestive heart failure. *Journal of the American Geriatrics Society, 48*(5 Suppl): S101-9.

psychological and existential states have been shown to improve Mount, B.M., Boston, P.H., & Cohen, S.R. (2007, April). Healing connections: On moving from suffering to a sense of well-being. *Journal of Pain and Symptom Management, 33*(4): 372–388, pp. 373–374.

48: loss of dignity or meaning Blinderman, C.D., & Cherny, N.I. (2005). Existential issues do not necessarily result in existential suffering: Lessons from cancer patients in Israel. *Palliative Medicine, 19*: 371–380.

dying people don't necessarily consider themselves sick Mount, B.M., Boston, P.H., & Cohen, S.R. (2007, April). Healing connections: On moving from suffering to a sense of well-being. *Journal of Pain and Symptom Management, 33*(4): 372–388, p. 373.

50: unfamiliar work Coyle, N. (2006, September). The hard work of living in the face of death. *Journal of Pain and Symptom Management, 32*(3): 266–274, p. 267.

it will choose to activate Howell, D., Fitch, M., & Deane, K. (2003). Impact of ovarian cancer perceived by women. *Cancer Nursing, 26*(1): 7.

51: their desire to prolong living Nissim, R., Rennie, D., Fleming, S., Hales, S., Gagliese, L., & Rodin, G. (2012). Goals set in the land of the living/dying: A longitudinal study of patients living with advanced cancer. *Death Studies, 36*: 360–390, p. 371.

it's like super gambling Nissim, R., Rennie, D., Fleming, S., Hales, S., Gagliese, L., & Rodin, G. (2012). Goals set in the land of the living/dying: A longitudinal study of patients living with advanced cancer. *Death Studies, 36*: 360–390, p. 371.

52: patients often went to still another set of doctors Nissim, R., Rennie, D., Fleming, S., Hales, S., Gagliese, L., & Rodin, G. (2012). Goals set in the land of the living/dying: A longitudinal study of patients living with advanced cancer. *Death Studies, 36*: 360–390, p. 370.

who was at fault Coyle, N. (2006, September). The hard work of living in the face of death. *Journal of Pain and Symptom Management, 32*(3): 266–274, p. 269.

53: we didn't fight for a long time Howell, D., Fitch, M.I., & Deane, K.A. (2003). Impact of ovarian cancer perceived by women. *Cancer Nursing, 26*(1): 1–9, p. 4.

how uncomfortable people are around cancer patients Howell, D., Fitch, M.I., & Deane, K.A. (2003). Impact of ovarian cancer perceived by women. *Cancer Nursing, 26*(1): 1–9, p. 7.

no two ways about it Howell, D., Fitch, M.I., & Deane, K.A. (2003). Impact of ovarian cancer perceived by women. *Cancer Nursing, 26*(1): 1–9, p. 4.

cancer patients receive more social support Tempelaar, R., De Haes, J.C., De Ruiter, J.H., Bakker, D., Van Den Heuvel, W.J., & Van Nieuwenhuijzen, M.G. (1989). The social experiences of cancer under treatment: A comparative study. *Social Science Medicine, 29*(5): 635–642.

54: allowing others to support and care for us Byock, I. (2004, 2014). *The four things that matter most: A book about living* (p. 94). New York: Atria Books.

CHAPTER FOUR: GOING HOME: WHERE PEOPLE DIE

58: while about 80 percent of Americans Centers for Disease Control and Prevention, National Center for Health Statistics. Underlying cause of death 1999-2016 on CDC WONDER Online Database, released December 2017. Retrieved April 28, 2018, from wonder.cdc.gov/ucd-icd10.html.

69 he was more likely to die in a hospital Pritchard, R.S., Fisher, E., Teno, J.M., & Lynn, J. (1998, October). Influence of patient preferences and local health system characteristics on the place of death. *Journal of the American Geriatrics Society, 46*(10): 1242–1250.

63: they wanted to die at home but ended up dying in a hospital Srivastava, R. (2017, May 1). Dying at home might sound preferable. But I've seen the reality. *The Guardian.*

64: end of life care by professionals Thomas, C., Morris, S.M., & Clark, D. (2004). Place of death: Preferences among cancer patients and their carers. *Social Science & Medicine, 58*: 2431–2444, p. 2439.

70 percent for patients Flory, J., Young-Xu, Y., Gurol, I., Levinsky, N., Ash, A., & Emanuel, E. (2004, May). Place of death: U.S. trends since 1980. *Health Affairs, 23*(3): 194–200.

the number has since dropped Bekelman, J., Halpern, S.D., Blankart, C.R., Bynum, J.P., Cohen, J., Fowler, R., . . . & Emanuel, E.J. (2016, January 19). Comparison of site of death, health care utilization, and hospital expenditures for patients dying with cancer in 7 developed countries. *Journal of the American Medical Association, 315*(3): 272–283, p. 272.

65: Medicare is the primary payer for 85 percent National Hospice and Palliative Care Organization. (2018,

March). NHPCO facts and figures: Hospice care in America. Alexandria, VA. Retrieved February 8, 2017, from www.nhpco .org/sites/default/files/public/Statistics_Research/2017_Facts _Figures.pdf

67: forty percent of hospice patients use the service for two weeks or less National Hospice and Palliative Care Organization. (2018, March). NHPCO facts and figures: Hospice care in America. Alexandria, VA. Retrieved February 8, 2017, from www.nhpco.org/sites/default/files/public/Statistics _Research/2017_Facts_Figures.pdf.

family members were twice as likely to rate care Teno, J.M., Freedman, V.A., Kasper, J.D., Gozalo, P., & Mor, V. (2015). Is care for the dying improving in the United States? *Journal of Palliative Medicine, 18*(8): 662–666, p. 665.

73: 70 percent of hospices in the United States are now home based Baxter, A. (2017, October 8). What hospice care looks like in America. *Home Health Care News.* Retrieved March 6, 2018, from homehealthcarenews.com/2017/10/what -hospice-care-looks-like-in-america.

their families' needs were met better Teno, J.M., Clarridge, B.R., Casey, V., Welch, L.C., Wetle, T., Shield, R., & Mor, V. (2004, January 7). Family perspectives on end-of-life care at the last place of care. *Journal of the American Medical Association, 291*(1): 88–93, p. 91.

the sheer hard work of dying Pollock, K. (2015, October). Is home always the best and preferred place of death? *The BMJ, 7*(351): 1–3, p. 1.

74: end-of-life care can evolve Bekelman, J., Halpern, S.D., Blankart, C.R., Bynum, J.P., Cohen, J., Fowler, R., . . . & Emanuel, E.J. (2016, January 19). Comparison of site of death, health care utilization, and hospital expenditures for patients dying with cancer in 7 developed countries. *Journal of the American Medical Association, 315*(3): 272–283, p. 280.

three or more hospitalizations in the last ninety days

of life Teno, J.M., Gozalo, P.L., Bynum, J.P.W., Leland, N.E., Miller, S.C., Morden, N.E., . . . & Mor, V. (2013, February 6). Change in end-of-life care for Medicare beneficiaries: Site of death, place of care, and health care transitions in 2000, 2005, and 2009. *Journal of the American Medical Association, 309*(5): 470–477, p. 474.

74: the number of moves in the last seventy-two hours of patients' Teno, J.M., Freedman, V.A., Kasper, J.D., Gozalo, P., & Mor, V. (2015). Is care for the dying improving in the United States? *Journal of Palliative Medicine, 18*(8): 662–666, p. 665.

the number of people dying in nursing homes Teno, J.M., Clarridge, B.R., Casey, V., Welch, L.C., Wetle, T., Shield, R., & Mor, V. (2004, January 7). Family perspectives on end-of-life care at the last place of care. *Journal of the American Medical Association, 291*(1): 88–93, p. 92.

75: most appropriate and desired Tang, S.T. (2003). When death is imminent: Where terminally ill patients with cancer prefer to die and why. *Cancer Nursing, 26*(3): 245–251, p. 249.

76: Medicare will help to pay the costs Aragon, K., Covinsky, K., Miao, Y., Boscardin, W.J., Flint, L., & Smith, A.K. (2012, November 12). Use of the Medicare posthospitalization skilled nursing benefit in the last 6 months of life. *Archives of Internal Medicine, 172*(20): 1573–1579, p. 1573.

the nursing home has a more homelike Tang, S.T. (2003). When death is imminent: Where terminally ill patients with cancer prefer to die and why. *Cancer Nursing, 26*(3): 245–251, p. 248.

77: I hope I don't need that Thomas, C., Morris, S.M., & Clark, D. (2004). Place of death: Preferences among cancer patients and their carers. *Social Science & Medicine, 58:* 2431–2444, p. 2440.

more likely to have untreated pain Teno, J.M., Clarridge, B.R., Casey, V., Welch, L.C., Wetle, T., Shield, R., & Mor, V.

(2004, January 7). Family perspectives on end-of-life care at the last place of care. *Journal of the American Medical Association, 291*(1): 88–93, p. 91.

78: most people would prefer, presumably, to be not ill Pollock, K. (2015, October). Is home always the best and preferred place of death? *The BMJ, 7*(351): 1–3, p. 2.

the unfathomable experience of dying Pollock, K. (2015, October). Is home always the best and preferred place of death? *The BMJ, 7*(351): 1–3, p. 2.

CHAPTER FIVE: DOES DYING HURT?

81: the experience of dying in the United States has grown worse Teno, J.M., Freedman, V.A., Kasper, J.D., Gozalo, P., & Mor, V. (2015). Is care for the dying improving in the United States? *Journal of Palliative Medicine, 18*(8): 662–666.

researchers interviewed family members from 1998 to 2010 Singer, A.E., Meeker, D., Teno, J.M., Lynn, J., Lunney, J.R., & Lorenz, K.A. (2015). Symptom trends in the last year of life from 1998 to 2010: A cohort study. *Annals of Internal Medicine, 162*(3): 175–188.

82: that 50 percent reported moderate or serious pain Weiss, S.C., Emanuel, L.L., Fairclough, D.L., & Emanuel, E.J. (2001, April 28). Understanding the experience of pain in terminally ill patients. *The Lancet, 357*: 1311–1314, p. 1311.

83: the images in our mind are extraordinarily rich Gawande, A. (2008, June 30). The itch: Its mysterious power may be a clue to a new theory about brains and bodies. *The New Yorker*. Retrieved September 8, 2017, from www.newyorker.com/magazine/2008/06/30/the-itch.

84: pain is always subjective IASP Terminology. (2017, December 14). In International Association for the Study of Pain. Retrieved April 29, 2018, from www.iasp-pain.org/Education /Content.aspx?ItemNumber=1698.

84: an experience embedded in beliefs about causes and diseases Cassell, E.J. (1991, 2004). *The nature of suffering and the goals of medicine* (p. 267). New York: Oxford University Press.

85: amputation was not in anybody's thoughts Cassell, E.J. (1991, 2004). *The nature of suffering and the goals of medicine* (p. 269). New York: Oxford University Press.

pain is not suffering Cassell, E.J. (1991, 2004). *The nature of suffering and the goals of medicine* (p. xii). New York: Oxford University Press.

when they feel out of control Cassell, E.J. (1991, 2004). *The nature of suffering and the goals of medicine* (p. 35). New York: Oxford University Press.

86: perhaps the most intractable pain of all Clark, D. (Ed.). (2006). Introduction. In *Cicely Saunders: Selected writings 1958-2004* (pp. xiii–xxviii). Oxford, UK: Oxford University Press.

87: I accepted the pain Coyle, N. (2006, September). The hard work of living in the face of death. *Journal of Pain and Symptom Management, 32*(3): 266–274.

89: morphine is so often prescribed to dying people Flemming, K. (2010, January). The use of morphine to treat cancer-related pain: A synthesis of quantitative and qualitative research. *Journal of Pain and Symptom Management, 39*(1): 139–154.

115 people a day die from an opioid overdose National Institute on Drug Abuse. (2018, March). Opioid overdose crisis. Retrieved May 10, 2018, from www.drugabuse.gov/drugs-abuse/opioids/opioid-overdose-crisis#one.

90: the frightening spread in street use Meldrum, M.L. (2003, November 12). A capsule history of pain management. *Journal of the American Medical Association, 290*(18): 2470–2475, p. 2471.

addiction is rarely an issue Fine, R.L. (2007, January).

Ethical and practical issues with opioids in life-limiting illness. *Proceedings of Baylor University Medical Center, 20*(1): 5–12.
96: short-circuited or prevented De Graeff, A., & Dean, M. (2007). Palliative sedation therapy in the last weeks of life: A literature review and recommendations for standards. *Journal of Palliative Medicine, 10*(1): 67–85, p. 71.
98: own personal limits of endurance Clark, D. (Ed.). (2002). *Cicely Saunders: Founder of the hospice movement, selected letters 1959-1999* (p. 17). New York: Oxford University Press.

CHAPTER SIX: COPING: A MAP FOR HOW TO DIE WELL

101: the best time we have ever spent together Byock, I. (1997). *Dying well: Peace and possibilities at the end of life* (p. 30). New York: Riverhead Books.
good deaths were not random events Byock, I. (1997). *Dying well: Peace and possibilities at the end of life* (p. 31). New York: Riverhead Books.
102: many patients seem to cope effectively Weisman, A., & Worden, J.W. (1976). The existential plight in cancer: Significance of the first 100 days. *International Journal of Psychiatry in Medicine, 7*(1): 1–15, p. 2.
103: she is so alive Clark, D. (Ed.). (2006). *Cicely Saunders: Selected writings 1958-2004* (pp. 129–130). Oxford, UK: Oxford University Press.
what they have done to our thoughts on death Clark, D. (Ed.). (2006). *Cicely Saunders: Selected writings 1958-2004* (p. 130). Oxford, UK: Oxford University Press.
105: people find little guidance Lynn, J. (2005). Living long in fragile health: The new demographics shape end of life care. *Hastings Center Report,* Nov.-Dec. Spec. No. S14-18, p. S14.

105: nobody teaches you Coyle, N. (2006, September). The hard work of living in the face of death. *Journal of Pain and Symptom Management, 32*(3): 266–274, p. 267.

106: refuse to acknowledge more than a minimum about illness Weisman, A., & Worden, J.W. (1976). The existential plight in cancer: Significance of the first 100 days. *International Journal of Psychiatry in Medicine, 7*(1): 1–15, p. 12.

they may share worries with others Weisman, A., & Worden, J.W. (1976). The existential plight in cancer: Significance of the first 100 days. *International Journal of Psychiatry in Medicine, 7*(1): 1–15, p. 12.

111: the process of dying is rarely enjoyable Byock, I. (1997). *Dying well: Peace and possibilities at the end of life* (p. 218). New York: Riverhead Books.

112: there is no 'good' way to cope Wrubel, J., Acree, M., Goodman S., & Folkman, S. (2009, December). End of living: Maintaining a lifeworld during terminal illness. *Psychology and Health, 24*(10): 1229–1243, p. 1239.

express anger and frustration Wrubel, J., Acree, M., Goodman S., & Folkman, S. (2009, December). End of living: Maintaining a lifeworld during terminal illness. *Psychology and Health, 24*(10): 1229–1243, p. 1238.

114: nobody is looking at him as a person Nissim, R., Freeman, E., Lo, C., Zimmermann, C., Gagliese, L., Rydall, A., . . . & Rodin, G. (2011). Managing cancer and living meaningfully (CALM): A qualitative study of a brief individual psychotherapy for individuals with advanced cancer. *Palliative Medicine, 26*(5): 713–721, p. 718.

115: I actually don't want them to help Nissim, R., Freeman, E., Lo, C., Zimmermann, C., Gagliese, L., Rydall, A., . . . & Rodin, G. (2011). Managing cancer and living meaningfully (CALM): A qualitative study of a brief individual psychotherapy for individuals with advanced cancer. *Palliative Medicine, 26*(5): 713–721, p. 717.

117: unspoken taboo Nissim, R., Freeman, E., Lo, C., Zimmermann, C., Gagliese, L., Rydall, A., ... & Rodin, G. (2011). Managing cancer and living meaningfully (CALM): A qualitative study of a brief individual psychotherapy for individuals with advanced cancer. *Palliative Medicine, 26*(5): 713–721, p. 716.

CHAPTER SEVEN: GROWTH AND LEGACIES

124: her dying had become the very means of her growth Clark, D. (Ed.). (2006). *Cicely Saunders: Selected writings 1958-2004* (p. 130). Oxford, UK: Oxford University Press.

have the capacity to change Byock, I. (2004, 2014). *The four things that matter most: A book about living* (p. 26). New York: Atria Books.

127: great good can come from great suffering Tedeschi, R., & Calhoun, L. (2004). Posttraumatic growth: Conceptual foundations and empirical evidence. *Psychological Inquiry, 15*(1): 1–18, p. 1.

the experience of positive change Tedeschi, R., & Calhoun, L. (2004). Posttraumatic growth: Conceptual foundations and empirical evidence. *Psychological Inquiry, 15*(1): 1–18, p. 1.

experience some growth Calhoun, L., & Tedeschi, R. (2013). *Posttraumatic growth in clinical practice* (p. 13). New York: Routledge.

the evidence is overwhelming Tedeschi, R., & Calhoun, L. (2004). Posttraumatic growth: Conceptual foundations and empirical evidence. *Psychological Inquiry, 15*(1): 1–18, p. 3.

truly traumatic circumstances Tedeschi, R., & Calhoun, L. (2004). Posttraumatic growth: Conceptual foundations and empirical evidence. *Psychological Inquiry, 15*(1): 1–18, pp. 1–2.

128: the whole idea of posttraumatic growth Calhoun, L.G., & Tedeschi, R.G. (2004). The foundations of posttraumatic growth: New considerations. *Psychological Inquiry, 15*(1): 93–102, p. 98.

I am a more sensitive person Kushner, H.S. (1981). *When bad things happen to good people* (p. 147). New York: Anchor Books.

130: I can live through just about anything Calhoun, L., & Tedeschi, R. (2013). *Posttraumatic growth in clinical practice* (p. 7). New York: Routledge.

close friendships between the man and some of his colleagues Calhoun, L., & Tedeschi, R. (2013). *Posttraumatic growth in clinical practice* (p. 9). New York: Routledge.

I am permanently wounded Calhoun, L., & Tedeschi, R. (2013). *Posttraumatic growth in clinical practice* (p. 2). New York: Routledge.

131: more likely to experience posttraumatic growth Barskova, T., & Oesterreich, R. (2009). Post-traumatic growth in people living with a serious medical condition and its relations to physical and mental health: A systematic review. *Disability and Rehabilitation, 31*(21): 1709–1733.

survive their struggles Tedeschi, R., & Calhoun, L. (2004). Posttraumatic growth: Conceptual foundations and empirical evidence. *Psychological Inquiry, 15*(1): 1–18, p. 15.

the trauma was so overwhelming Tang, S.T., Lin, K.C., Chen, J.S., Chang, W.C., Hsieh, C.H., & Chou, W.C. (2015). Threatened with death but growing: Changes in and determinants of posttraumatic growth over the dying process for Taiwanese terminally ill cancer patients. *Psycho-Oncology, 24*: 147–154.

more rewarding relationships See, for example, Widows, M.R., Jacobsen, P.B., Booth-Jones, M., & Fields, K.K. (2005). Predictors of posttraumatic growth following bone marrow transplantation for cancer. *Health Psychology, 24*(3): 266–273;

Schulz, U., & Mohamed, N.E. (2004). Turning the tide: Benefit finding after cancer. *Social Science & Medicine, 59*: 653–662; Mystakidou, K., Tsilika, E., Parpa, E., Kyriakopoulos, D., Malamos, N., & Damigos, D. (2008). Personal growth and psychological distress in advanced breast cancer. *The Breast,* 17: 382–386; and Taylor, E.J. (2000). Transformation of tragedy among women surviving breast cancer. *Oncology Nursing Forum, 27*(5): 781–788, p. 786.

132: appreciate what you have right now Taylor, E.J. (2000). Transformation of tragedy among women surviving breast cancer. *Oncology Nursing Forum, 27*(5): 781–788, p. 786.

why are we here Mount, B.M., Boston, P.H., & Cohen, S.R. (2007, April). Healing connections: On moving from suffering to a sense of well-being. *Journal of Pain and Symptom Management, 33*(4): 372–388, p. 378.

a chance to evolve spiritually Mount, B.M., Boston, P.H., & Cohen, S.R. (2007, April). Healing connections: On moving from suffering to a sense of well-being. *Journal of Pain and Symptom Management, 33*(4): 372–388, p. 379.

135: a surrender to the transcendent Byock, I. (1996). The nature of suffering and the nature of opportunity at the end of life. *Clinics in Geriatric Medicine, 12*(2): 237–252, p. 248.

136: they all describe themselves as spiritual in some way Byock, I. (2008). Personal growth and human development in life-threatening conditions: Therapeutic insights and strategies derived from positive experiences of individuals and families. In H. Chochinov & W. Breitbart (Eds.), *Handbook of Psychiatry in Palliative Medicine* (pp. 281–299). Oxford: Oxford University Press.

140: the only person who can tell the story is that individual Chochinov, H. (2016, September 1). Dignity therapy. [Video File.] Retrieved August 20, 2017, from www.youtube.com/watch?v=ZHOteLkTdeU.

140: I feel intensely alive Sacks, O. (2015, February 19). My own life. *New York Times*. Retrieved July 6, 2017, from www .nytimes.com.

we see people go through a lifetime of experience Clark, D. (Ed.). 2006. *Cicely Saunders: Selected writings 1958-2004* (pp. 130–131). Oxford, UK: Oxford University Press.

CHAPTER EIGHT: CHECKING OUT EARLY

151: peaceful, with little suffering Schwarz, J. (2011). Death by voluntary dehydration: Suicide or the right to refuse a life-prolonging measure? *Widener Law Review, 17*(351): 351–361, p. 357.

152: patients have received lethal prescriptions Oregon Public Health Division, Center for Health Statistics. (2018, February 9). Oregon Death with Dignity Act: Data Summary 2017, p. 5. Retrieved May 17, 2018, from www.oregon.gov.

155: 47 percent or fewer of surveyed physicians supported aid in dying Emanuel, E.J., Onwuteaka-Philpsen, B.D., Urwin, J.W., & Cohen, J. (2016). Attitudes and practices of euthanasia and physician-assisted suicide in the United States, Canada, and Europe. *Journal of the American Medical Association, 316*(1): 79–90, p. 81.

CHAPTER NINE: THE BRAIN AND DYING

167: awake and alert two weeks before death Morita, T., Ichiki, T., Tsunoda, J., Inoue, S., & Chihara, S. (1998, July/August). A prospective study on the dying process in terminally ill cancer patients. *The American Journal of Hospice & Palliative Care, 15*(4): 217–222, p. 220.

remain conscious until the very end of life Lichter, I., & Hunt, E. (1990). The last 48 hours of life. *Journal of Palliative Care, 6*(4): 7–15.

medications often make patients less alert See, for instance, reports of terminal cancer patients on opioids in Morita, T., Ichiki, T., Tsunoda, J., Inoue, S., & Chihara, S. (1998, July/August). A prospective study on the dying process in terminally ill cancer patients. *The American Journal of Hospice & Palliative Care, 15*(4): 217–222, p. 220; and Lichter, I., & Hunt, E. (1990). The last 48 hours of life. *Journal of Palliative Care, 6*(4): 7–15, p. 8.

168: a corresponding increase in cognitive impairment Bruera, E., Macmillan, K., Hanson, J., & MacDonald, R.N. (1989, October). The cognitive effects of the administration of narcotic analgesics in patients with cancer pain. *Pain, 39*(1): 13–16.

many of these patients are less alert Clemons, M., Regnard, C., & Appleton, T. (1996). Alertness, cognition and morphine in patients with advanced cancer. *Cancer Treatment Reviews, 22*: 451–468.

171–72: new ways of testing for responses Monti, M.M., Vanhaudenhuyse, A., Coleman, M.R., Boly, M., Pickard, J. D., Tshibanda, L., . . . & Laureys, S. (2010, February 10). Willful modulation of brain activity in disorders of consciousness. *New England Journal of Medicine, 362*(7): 579–589.

172: imagining the activity that corresponded Monti, M.M., Vanhaudenhuyse, A., Coleman, M.R., Boly, M., Pickard, J.D., Tshibanda, L., . . . & Laureys, S. (2010, February 10). Willful modulation of brain activity in disorders of consciousness. *New England Journal of Medicine, 362*(7): 579–589, p. 585.

173: minimally conscious patients hear their own names Perrin, F., Schnakers, C., Schabus, M., Degueldre, C., Goldman, S., Brédart, S., . . . & Laureys, S. (2006, April). Brain response to one's own name in vegetative state, minimally conscious state, and locked-in syndrome. *Archives of Neurology, 63*: 562–569.

173: retain some language recognition See Naro, A., Leo, A., Cannavò A., Buda, A., Bramanti, P., & Calabrò R.S. (2016, March). Do unresponsive wakefulness syndrome patients feel pain? Role of laser-evoked potential-induced gamma-band oscillations in detecting cortical pain processing. *Neuroscience, 317*: 141–148; Boly, M., Faymonville, M.E., Schnakers, C., Peigneux, P., Lambermont, B., Phillips, C., . . . & Laureys, S. (2008, November). Perception of pain in the minimally conscious state with PET activation: An observational study. *The Lancet Neurology, 11*: 1013–1020; and Coleman, M.R., Rodd, J.M., Davis, M.H., Johnsrude, I.S., Menon, D.K., Pickard, J.D., & Owen, A.M. (2007). Do vegetative patients retain aspects of language comprehension? Evidence from fMRI. *Brain, 130*: 2494–2507.

177: hospice patients may experience delirium Alici, Y., & Breitbart, W. (2009, May). Delirium in palliative care. *Primary Psychiatry, 16*(5): 42–48, p. 43.

178: because of frightening hallucinations or delusions Breitbart, W., Gibson, C., & Tremblay, A. (2002, May-June). The delirium experience: Delirium recall and delirium-related distress in hospitalized patients with cancer, their spouses/caregivers, and their nurses. *Psychosomatics 43*(3): 183–194, p. 188.

182: the dying patients' dreams were more intense Kerr, C.W., Donnelly, J.P., Wright, S.T., Kuszczak, S.M., Banas, A., Grant, P.C., & Luczkiewicz, D.L. (2014). End-of-life dreams and visions: A longitudinal study of hospice patients' experiences. *Journal of Palliative Medicine, 17*(3): 296–303, p. 302.

CHAPTER TEN: THE LAST FEW HOURS

186: we speak of 'death agonies' Nuland, S. B. (1993/1995). *How we die: Reflections on life's final chapter* (p. 121). New York: Vintage Books.

188: mostly by being overly optimistic See Christakis, N.A., & Lamont, E.B. (2000, February 19). Extent and determinants of error in doctors' prognoses in terminally ill patients: A prospective cohort study. *The BMJ, 320*(7233): 469–473; and Glare, P., Virik, K., Jones, M., Hudson, M., Eychmuller, S., Simes, J., & Christakis, N. (2003, July 26). A systematic review of physicians' survival predictions in terminally ill cancer patients. *The BMJ, 327*(7408): 195–198, p. 215.

193: death can be a messy experience Campbell, M.L., & Yarandi, H.N. (2013). Death rattle is not associated with patient respiratory distress: Is pharmacologic treatment indicated? *Journal of Palliative Medicine, 16*(10): 1255–1259.

194: mental and physical pain usually recede Clark, D. (Ed.). (2006). *Cicely Saunders: Selected writings 1958-2004* (p. 32). Oxford, UK: Oxford University Press.

no conclusive studies have determined the cause Plonk, W.M., & Armold, R.M. (2005). Terminal care: The last weeks of life. *Journal of Palliative Medicine, 8*(5): 1042–1054.

the final days leading up to that moment Lichter, I., & Hunt, E. (1990). The last 48 hours of life. *Journal of Palliative Care, 6*(4): 7–15.

195: patients certainly do die peacefully Lichter, I., & Hunt, E. (1990). The last 48 hours of life. *Journal of Palliative Care, 6*(4): 7–15, p. 7.

196: first hunger and then thirst are lost Hallenbeck, J. (2003). *Palliative Care Perspectives* (p. 220). New York: Oxford University Press.

197: most did not experience hunger at all McCann, R.M., Hall, W.J., & Groth-Juncker, A.G. (1994, October 26). Comfort care for terminally ill patients: The appropriate use of nutrition and hydration. *Journal of the American Medical Association, 272*(16): 1263–1266.

while dying people are often thirsty Ellershaw, J.E.,

Sutcliffe, J.M., & Saunders, C.M. (1995, April). Dehydration and the dying patient. *Journal of Pain and Symptom Management, 10*(3): 192–197.

197–98: patients' ability to engage in complex communications Morita, T., Tei, Y., & Inoue, S. (2003, September). Impaired communication capacity and agitated delirium in the final week of terminally ill cancer patients: Prevalence and identification of research focus. *Journal of Pain and Symptom Management, 26*(3): 827–834.

acknowledgments

A few people who work with the dying have told me they no longer fear their own deaths. I don't know whether that's true for me; I do know these are professionals whom I would trust—will trust—as I'm dying. They are an exceptionally caring group. At each stage of this project, there have been people who took a leap of faith to help it along the way.

Thanks to Pat Amthor, the Durango hospice nurse, for her frankness so many years ago about my mother's dying process. Thanks to David Hui, one of the first people I interviewed for this book, for his patience; to Margaret Campbell, who was so encouraging as I first began my research, and to Virginia Lee at McGill University, Céline Gélinas, David Hovda, and Nessa Coyle—all wonderful scholars whose care and thoroughness have been inspiring.

Thanks to Paul Bisceglio at The Atlantic.com, who recognized early on the importance of the subject and whose editing has been so consistently skillful. Thanks to my agent, Jane Dystel, and her associate agent, Miriam Goderich, without whom this book might not have seen the light of day. Thanks to the sensitive editing of Denise Silvestro at Kensington.

Thanks to Faron Scott, with whom I first learned about

writing and publishing a book. I'll always be grateful for our friendship.

Thanks to Mac Johnson in Durango for his generosity in speaking with me when his wife was dying.

Thanks to Joan Teno and Joanne Lynn, who study systemic trends and thereby help not just individuals but thousands of people.

Thanks to James Hallenbeck and Lonny Shavelson, who each set aside significant portions of a day to explain their work to me. Thanks to Scott Podolsky and David S. Jones, both of whom showed an especially delightful intellectual enthusiasm.

Thanks to Gary Rodin, Harvey Chochinov, and James Bernat for the amount of time and care they took in interpreting their research for me. Thanks to Kevin Nelson, who left a meeting early in order to patiently answer my questions on a busy day.

Thanks to Ira Byock, who has written his own wonderful books about dying, for being so generous with his time and expertise.

Thanks to Peter Rogatz, Laurie Leonard, Fred Schwartz, Judith Schwarz, Sue Dessayer Porter, Terry Law, and Barbara Sarah, all of whom have done so much to help dying people.

Thanks to Emery Brown at Harvard University, and to Jeremy Brown at the National Institutes of Health. Thanks to Marian Grant and Nick Martin, both of the Coalition to Transform Advanced Care.

Thanks to Hospice of Mercy, and its many staff members who have been so gracious both to their patients and to me. Not only did they welcome me into their meetings, but several—Michelle Appenzeller, Crystal Harris, Sean Kelly, Anne Rossignol, and Deb Callahan—sat for interviews, doing their best to answer my many questions. Other staff members have offered me extra support or thoughtful advice along the way: Erica Kelly, Miko Ketchin, Sherri Guyette, Sherrie Cayton.

And thanks to the hospice patients, who have so often taught me through example: some through their frankness about how much they were frustrated or pained by the experience of dying; some through the ways they rose to meet the challenges in front of them; some in the quiet ways they suffered or expressed a sense of joy or peace.

As I was finishing the edits on this book, the Zen Hospice Guest House in San Francisco closed its doors, and in doing so, ended an era of a particular kind of gracious aid to dying people. I'm grateful to have witnessed that hospitality. Thanks to Roy Remer, the former volunteer coordinator, for not saying no when I called out of the blue and asked to come train and then volunteer at the Guest House. Thanks to MaryEllen Kirkpatrick, the Guest House chef, whose Buddhist practices helped create a tranquil and orderly kitchen, and who put me up at her home for part of my stay. Thanks to the many other volunteers and staff members who made me feel so welcome there. And thanks to the San Francisco Zen Center, which provided a convenient and peaceful place for me to stay each of the times I volunteered at the Guest House, and where so many interesting and kind-hearted people reside.

Thanks in memory of Frank A. Lederle, who sent me a copy of the essay he wrote about his own experience with a terminal disease. Thanks to the many, many patients who unknowingly taught me so much.

Thanks to Caroline Arlen, whose early edits on a few key chapter drafts were so helpful. Thanks to Chris Goold, who listened to me and offered so much positive encouragement. Thanks to Sydney and Mitch Dion, who listened to early drafts as I read them aloud under the stars or over camp coffee, and offered me their ideas and gentle critiques. And to

June Tanner, whom I first met when she was a hospice patient and who has become a friend.

Thanks to all the Dears—Walt, Elizabeth, Bryan, Jacquelyn, Tristan, and Kalen—who have been supportive and encouraging, no matter how crazy the effort must have seemed at times.

And finally, I wish for all writers that they could have a champion like Tom Bartels, my first and best reader.